LIVING
MIRACLES

LIVING

MIRACLES

Stories of Hope from Parents

of Premature Babies

KIMBERLY A. POWELL

& KIM WILSON, Editors

Foreword by Jeffrey Thompson, M.D.

ST. MARTIN'S PRESS ✹ NEW YORK

Grateful acknowledgment is given to the parents whose stories are recounted here and reprinted, along with photographs, by permission.

Information in the glossary is derived from *The Premature Baby Book: A Parents' Guide to Coping and Caring in the First Years* by Helen Harrison and Ann Kositsky, R.N. Copyright © 1983 by Helen Harrison. Reprinted by permission of St. Martin's Press, LLC.

Library of Congress Cataloging-in-Publication Data

Living miracles : stories of hope from parents of premature babies / Kimberly A. Powell and Kim Wilson [editors].—1st ed.
    p. cm.
    ISBN 0-312-24550-5
    1. Infants (Premature)—Popular works. 2. Birth weight, Low—Complications—Popular works. 3. Parents—Attitudes. I. Powell, Kimberly A. II. Wilson, Kimberly.
RJ250.L57 2000
618.92′011—dc21   99-089725

Book designed by Michelle McMillian

First Edition: April 2000

10 9 8 7 6 5 4 3 2 1

For Dustin and Senia,
heroes, sources of inspiration,
and our living miracles

A NOTE TO READERS

CONTENTS

Samuel was born at 1 pound 8 ounces when his mother went into pre-term labor. His parents had endured infertility treatments and miscarriages for more than nine years. While Samuel has some speech delays and swallowing problems, he is rapidly improving and is a happy two-and-a-half-year-old.

At 1 pound 5 ounces Anna entered the world early due to fetal growth retardation. While it is still too early to tell if Anna will have long-term developmental obstacles, at two and a half years old she appreciates life more than most. No one who knows Anna's story would bet against her.

Now four years old, Austin and Ashli beat the odds to survive premature labor, surgeries, and low birth weight. Austin was 1 pound 8

odds. He is now one year old and has some minor delays in gross-motor skills, speech, and fine-motor skills. Trace's parents can't believe they have been so blessed and cannot imagine their lives without him.

Orvin Bakken entered this world in 1921 weighing 1 pound 4 ounces. Relying on instinct and prayer, his mother nurtured and cared for him at home in rural Iowa without the assistance of an NICU.

After preterm labor and sixty-three days in the Special Care Nursery, Megan is a very lucky preemie who did not suffer any of the serious problems that preemies are prone to. She was 2 pounds 8 ounces at birth.

A grandmother's poem.

The father of a preemie born three months early expresses the shock, disappointment, and anger often experienced by parents of preemies.

When a seemingly perfect pregnancy came to an abrupt end due to HELLP syndrome, Senia had to fight for her life. Starting at 1 pound 15 ounces, Senia came home on the one-year anniversary of her late grandfather's death—a sign that life is precious. At two years old, Senia continues to be proof of the value of life.

One miscarriage, an autoimmune disorder, HELLP syndrome, and intrauterine growth retardation made Sarah's chances at life bleak. Once a 1 pound 12 ounce baby, she is now a healthy two-year-old who has given her parents an experience that has changed them forever.

29 WEEKS' GESTATION

Only 2 pounds 15 ounces at birth, Brayden continues every day to fight for a quality life. At ten months old his cerebral palsy, cortical blindness, bradycardias, and oral defensiveness don't hinder his perseverance and strength.

The stress of losing her father to cancer took its toll on Robin, and preterm labor brought Ryan into the world early. During the last two and a half years he has been through multiple surgeries and pneumonia, but he has made it and is doing well. Ryan is proof that one should never give up hope.

31 WEEKS' GESTATION

Griffin surprised everyone when he weighed in at 5 pounds, although nine weeks premature due to placenta previa. He surprised everyone again by going home after only twenty days in the hospital—a short stay for such an early baby. At two years old Griffin is still full of surprises and has his parents wrapped around his tiny finger.

At four years old Noah is truly a miracle. After his mother developed HELLP syndrome, Noah entered the world early at 3 pounds 10 ounces. Many of Noah's challenges stemmed from VACTERLS syndrome, birth defects not related to prematurity but exacerbated by it. Noah's mother was told many times that he would die, but she never gave up on him and learned how precious life is and what a blessing children are.

32 WEEKS' GESTATION

PROM (premature rupture of membranes) is the cause for Dustin entering this world on a wing and a prayer. He amazed everyone by weighing in at 5 pounds 7.5 ounces. His serious battle for life began when he was thirteen days old and quit breathing in his grandmother's arms. After several bouts of apnea, bradycardia, and respiratory syncytial virus, he is now a cheerful, healthy six-year-old.

Due to a placental abruption brought on by pregnancy-induced hypertension, Mitchie entered the world eight weeks early, screaming his lungs out at 3 pounds 2.5 ounces. Mitchie survived one of the most dreaded preemie complications, necrotizing enterocolitis (NEC), and is now a happy, healthy four-year-old.

33 WEEKS' GESTATION

Rh incompatibility was thought to be the primary cause of Brayden's early arrival until the doctors performed a C-section and discovered the umbilical cord wrapped around his neck. After fighting and winning two life-threatening battles, Brayden is now an energetic, healthy eighteen-month-old.

35 WEEKS' GESTATION

Gestational diabetes contributed to the premature delivery of Aidan at 4 pounds 9 ounces. Once he learned to eat well, he went home and has no lasting evidence of his prematurity.

36 WEEKS' GESTATION

Bert Edens

When an amniocentesis revealed a rare chromosomal disorder, the Edenses were advised by numerous doctors to terminate the pregnancy. They refused, knowing they would love their child regardless of the outcome. A miracle in every way possible, Zak (Chigger) is now five years old and excited about starting kindergarten.

ACKNOWLEDGMENTS

Many people aided us in the preparation of this project.

I thank my daughter, Senia, for inspiring this book, showing me what strength really is, teaching me patience, and being the greatest gift of love I've ever received. I thank my husband, Larry Sikkink, for his love and sacrifice of time during this project; the late Glenn Sikkink as the inspiration for my living miracle; Louise Sikkink for her enthusiasm and eager questions through each stage of the book's conception; my parents, Madolyn and Ernest Powell, for their loving concern from Senia's birth through the publication of this book; my doctor, Karen Cowan, and the LaCrosse Gundersen Lutheran NICU nurses and doctors for their care of Senia, making her a living miracle; Dr. Jeffrey Thompson for writing the foreword and for help with the glossary; and Luther College for providing some financial assistance. Thanks to Carrie Niebur for her early contributions, and, finally, thanks to Rachel Faldet, Jyoti Grewal, and my friends, family, and colleagues for their support and interest in *Living Miracles*.

—K.A.P.

I thank first and foremost God. Without Him I never would have had my living miracle named Dustin or an interest in compiling this book. In addition, I want to thank my son, Dustin, for giving me inspiration and the opportunity to be a mom; and my husband, George, who always believed in this project—his constant encouragement and understanding will never be forgotten. I love you both. I also want to thank my family: Mom (Susie Lang), Dad (Kelly Lang), Jim, Dede, Sandy, and JR, along with my grandmothers, Darleen Bakken and Iva Nell Lang, and my numerous aunts and uncles. All of you have watched this book unfold since Dustin's birth in October 1993. You never gave up hope that it would be published. Thanks for your support and encouragement from the very beginning.

—K.W.

We both send a special thanks to Susie Lang for bringing us together to produce this book and for baby-sitting while we labored over it. We especially thank her for her never-ending belief that *Living Miracles* would be published because it was needed to provide hope to so many parents.

We also thank our agent, Meredith Bernstein, who worked enthusiastically to find the right publisher, and St. Martin's Press for being that publisher. Our editor at St. Martin's Press, Elizabeth Beier, and the entire production team deserve a special thanks for the final appearance of this book.

Finally, we extend a special thanks to all the parents who were willing to share their stories, for without them this book would not have been possible.

FOREWORD

The book you are about to read is a collection of intense stories straight from the heart. These parents describe in great detail the personal struggles of troubled pregnancies, endless days in the Neonatal Intensive Care Unit, and the myriad problems their infants faced after going home.

You will find specific information about the early stages of these far-from-storybook pregnancies. Some families struggle for months or years to establish a pregnancy. Mothers often take great risks in order to conceive and begin this adventure. Others find that despite careful planning and taking meticulous care of their diet, exercise, and stress levels, their body just does not cooperate. Although insensitive outsiders might imply that these mothers must have done something wrong, that is not usually the case. They do not deserve this, nor is it "fair." Rapid increases in blood pressure that develop during pregnancy continue to occur despite modern medicine's attempt to explain or control it. Certainly a mother cannot be blamed if the placenta chooses to implant over the cervix rather than the safer and more common position high on the upper uterine wall. The parents' stories are often made even more poignant by the descriptions of pregnant women trying to balance their own health with the well-being of their baby, their relationship with their spouses, and the children they have at home—all this as they are trying to maintain their sanity while being confined to a hospital bed or caring for themselves at home.

Once the child is delivered, the struggles are hardly over. A repeated theme in this book is the one-step-forward-several-steps-back battle that these young families face. These contributors go a long way toward helping you understand what it feels like to have a child going through these crises, and they consistently point out that you can't imagine what it is like until you have gone through it yourself. Some infants have minor respiratory problems that quickly resolve, others have severe problems that persist for weeks or months, or will plague them for the rest of their lives. Some extremely premature infants' lives hang in the balance for days on end. Other infants struggle with prematurity as well as the misfortune of being abnormally formed or missing important organs.

The triumph of these infants over these initial life-threatening barriers only gets them to the point of being challenged by a more subtle but no less dangerous array of problems. After struggling through a hostile intrauterine environment, tolerating the numerous procedures and treatments in the intensive care unit, and struggling to accomplish the very basic chores of breathing, eating, and keeping their heartbeat above 100, going home for these infants should be smooth sailing. But as you will see, despite their parents' pride and joy, this long-awaited trip home sometimes turns out to be brief. It culminates in a return to the hospital for apnea, gastroesophageal reflux, or respiratory syncytial virus bronchiolitis. For these families, it's great to have the baby at home but scary to face potentially life-threatening problems outside the environment that has nurtured the infant and family for weeks or even months. How do they do it? How do parents survive these struggles? One great reason is that while watching their infants' heroic struggle to breathe and survive, they feel that the least they can do is help them. Another driving force is hope. Often you'll hear parents say they "hope for the best but prepare for the worst." The "worst" happens, but not as often as most people think. The most easily collected numbers are whether the babies survive or not. But the baby's mental and neuromuscular facilities and the family's emotional intactness are important outcomes to measure as well.

The medical community's ability to keep smaller and smaller infants—and earlier and earlier premature infants—alive and well has steadily improved. Twenty years ago it was still common in some places that infants less than 1,000 grams or less than twenty-eight weeks of gestation were considered too small for treatment. Now infants twenty-four weeks of gestation and 650 grams have at least a 50 percent chance of survival in most instances. Infants at twenty-eight weeks of gestation have a closer to 90 percent chance of survival.

It is well known that those infants who have struggled through a hostile intrauterine environment and the difficulties of premature postnatal life are at great risk for mental difficulties. But *most* of these infants will function within the normal range. It is important to remember that although the statistics for a large group of patients are available, any individual patient comprises 100 percent of that family's and that child's experience. This collection shows that infants who appear to undergo similar struggles may experience remarkably different outcomes. Modern science often doesn't understand either why we turn out "okay" or why many of the problems that develop occur.

Like mental problems, neuromuscular problems (cerebral palsy, for example) are no less of an enigma. Although the incidence of severe difficulties following intracranial infections or remarkably low blood supply to parts of the brain is quite high, children without these risk factors also can end up with cerebral palsy. Some others with severe problems of this nature have normal neuromuscular activity. In a world that is fascinated with size, speed, and competitive advantage, these problems are particularly difficult for families and infants to cope with. While some patients brag about their child rolling over at three months, others are proud to have their child breathing on his own at three months or rolling over by seven or eight months. Focusing on your own child's accomplishments as opposed to competing with the rest of the world is a good lesson for parents of all infants.

The emotional struggles that are painfully recounted in this work are as long and arduous as any physical problem. Strife between parents, long-term depression, and even divorce are common among these struggling families. They struggle with the stress of intellectually knowing what is happening but emotionally not wanting to believe it is really happening to them. Anger at the situation is often directed at oneself, a spouse, or caregivers. And finally, repeatedly, the mothers will recount the persistent feeling that they, their bodies—that *something*—should have been different.

Woven into these stories are many wonderful lessons that can teach other families, medical caregivers, and family and friends of these precious little bundles. For the parents there are many themes of "never giving up hope," "hope overcoming fears," and of not isolating oneself from family and friends. Over and over again we'll hear that it is difficult to understand others unless we have gone through it, but how important it is that we make every effort to try. Another important lesson is that there is almost always someone in worse shape than you are. There will be a premature infant who has more problems, who is younger, who is sicker, whose parents have less support, who will struggle longer and harder or may not even survive to struggle long and hard. Another important message is that life is too precious to be caught up in minor things you can do nothing about. Getting excited about someone cutting in line at the grocery store or your favorite sports team losing seems quite minor compared to the Herculean struggles of these tiny people.

Healthcare providers will find an instance in every story where the family of the child could have been better supported, better educated, or better understood. Our obligation is to seek ways to understand the feelings and needs of these people in crisis and organize our care in a fashion that supports not only the technical medical needs but also the equally important emotional needs of these families. There are many poignant examples in this book of a single phrase or offhand comment that made a huge impact on a family when it was in shock, scared, or not completely comprehending the situation. This book will give you great insight into how healthcare providers attempt to help mothers and infants and how differently our intentions of doing good are often perceived.

This group of life stories will allow you to glimpse the stresses of troubled pregnancies, the arduous journey through a neonatal intensive care unit, and the joy, fear, and struggles of finally going home. The lessons to be learned are not subtle nor completely new. They're the age-old story of parents holding out hope for their infants, risking their own health for the well-being of their children, and leading the charge to ensure their child has the best possible outcome. It teaches us that feelings are more important than machines and a child is part of a unit that needs to be nourished and nurtured. It shows us that sometimes extraordinary efforts are required to accomplish the extraordinary success of a child surviving these struggles. It teaches us courage and persistence, that hope can be stronger than fear, and that the insurmountable can be surmounted. Here is this book's greatest truth. It is the unconditional love of a parent that is the strongest force these little miracles have going for them.

—Jeffrey Thompson, M.D.
Director of Neonatal Intensive Care
Gundersen Lutheran Hospital
La Crosse, Wisconsin

INTRODUCTION

While most parents have nine months to anticipate the birth of a baby, parents of premature babies have even less time to prepare for the inevitable roller coaster of emotions. We both have been pregnant and filled with anticipation of the birth of our first child. However, each of our pregnancies took unexpected turns, bringing them to premature ends. Kimberly Powell developed HELLP (hemolysis, elevated liver enzymes, and low blood platelets) syndrome and delivered a baby girl by emergency cesarean section, 1 pound 15 ounces and twelve weeks premature. Kim Wilson delivered a boy, 5 pounds 7½ ounces and eight weeks premature, due to PROM (premature rupture of membranes). Not knowing a soul in a similar situation, we each searched for books that would tell us what to expect and how to legitimize the emotions we were feeling, and provide hope that our babies could grow up "normal." We needed to read realistic, hopeful accounts that would help us survive the time in the hospital and afterward. Such a collection did not exist.

We first met when we began working on this book. Individually we saw the potential to help families struck by prematurity and were working on our own. Kim Powell had numerous conversations about prematurity with her daughter's day care provider, Susie Lang. Susie's grandson had also been premature, so they automatically connected, and Kim trusted her immediately with Senia. One day in

October 1997, Kim Powell was telling Susie about a book she was working on that would contain stories from parents of premature babies. Susie's eyes lit up as she said that her daughter, Kim Wilson, was working on the very same project. We spoke on the phone that evening and began working on this project together.

Living Miracles is designed to share how veteran parents of preemies cope, to ease fears, educate, and provide hope. While not all preemies survive and many have additional medical challenges, advancements in neonatology allow more preemies to survive and thrive than not. Those who have watched their premature baby fight for life know that preemies truly are living miracles.

THE PREEMIE EXPERIENCE

by Sandra D. Moore

*The preemie experience is the shattering of all your dreams
for a normal, healthy delivery,
of the ability to carry home a beautiful squirming bundle
after a short stay in the hospital.*

*It is lying there in your hospital room listening to
the happy sounds of whole families joined
together by the birth of a grandchild, cousin, niece,
or nephew, and knowing that your
child is miles away and may not survive long enough
for you to see or simply touch.*

*It is that first glimpse of a skinny, scrawny, not much bigger
than a Barbie doll child
and feeling fear, awe, and joy for such a fragile soul.*

*It is sitting by your baby's "bedside" day after day,
week after week, month after month,
alternating between the emotional high of "Look, her eyes
are open," or "She's crying!"
and the lows of "I'm sorry, Mrs. Moore. Something has
shown up in Lauren's ultrasound,"
or even "There is nothing we can do . . ."*

*It is hearing the alarms go off for the twentieth time in less
than fifteen minutes because your
child's heart rate keeps hitting zero.*

It is watching children dying around you, wondering if
your child will be next.

It is hearing your child's cry of distress as the nurses
insert yet another IV or do another
round of daily blood tests.

It is meeting other parents of children who are doing far better
and wondering, "Why me?"
And meeting parents of children who have just died
and praising God for His mercy
to your child and feeling guilty because your child is alive
and someone else is grieving for theirs.

It is days of nightmarish testing and coping with less
than positive results to the tests.

It is days of joy at seeing the first eyelash appear,
the child gain a whole ounce in one day,
and two bright shiny eyes look at you and into your soul,
and knowing that your child now recognizes you as Mama or Dada;
or perhaps looks at you and does not see you at all. . . .

It is that final hurdle before coming home!
It is the sorrow of waiting for the monitor company
representative to show you what to do
if the alarm sounds when your child is choking,
gasping for breath, or simply dying.
It is the joy of just being away from all those nurses
and tubes and wires and beeps, and
walking into the nursery you hastily prepared because, after all,
the child wasn't due for another three months!

It is thinking that the nightmare is over . . . only to realize that it still
continues in the form
of such acronyms as PVL, RSV, BPD, CP, and numerous others.

*It is the final realization that these developmental delays
have to be dealt with,
that reflux is a normal and unfortunate occurrence in most preemies,
that the constant fight to gain weight is in direct proportion
to a preemie's inability to do so.*

*It is watching a child struggle to pick up his or her head, sit,
crawl, or walk.
It is witnessing only silence when the child should be babbling,
because the child cannot hear.*

*It is the mental images of a child running and playing
and communicating with others in a
perfectly normal manner that are marred when you face years of therapy
in order to simply get the child to eat by himself or herself,
or talk or walk and then run.*

*The preemie experience is a journey . . .
a journey through your soul in order to find the faith and strength to cope,
a journey of the mind when you face the emotional weariness,
a journey of the heart . . . to accept that, no matter what,
this child is yours,
and you will love this child no matter what!*

LIVING

MIRACLES

INFERTILITY: A NINE-YEAR JOURNEY FOR SAMUEL

by Susan-Adelle Wilshire Warren

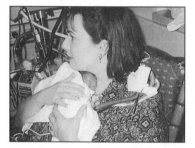

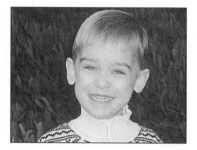

Samuel, one month old, being kangarood
by his mom, Susan, for the very first time.

Samuel, three years old.

Our nine-year journey of infertility actually started almost five years before we were married, in 1982, when I was eighteen years old and a freshman in college. I lived through toxic shock syndrome (TSS) acquired from using the super tampons made in the early 1980s. I had severe peritonitis and nearly died. Months later, after recovering and reenrolling in college, my appendix ruptured. This was misdiagnosed as a TSS relapse. The ruptured appendix stayed in my abdomen for days and wasn't discovered until they scheduled a laparotomy to clean out my bowels and remove my ovaries and uterus. A female surgeon refused to remove my reproductive organs (the head surgeon walked out of surgery at this point), but I was later told that I had little or no chance of having children.

Fast-forward to 1986. I graduated from college with a biology/chemistry degree and soon married my wonderful husband, a teacher whom I had met while singing in the church college choir. Within months of our marriage we started trying to conceive by charting basal body temperature and using ovulation prediction kits. After two years without success, we sought the help of infertility medicine. We had the full barrage of tests. The scarring from the abdominal infections had ruined one fallopian tube, and I found out I also had polycystic ovarian syndrome. We started with months of the fertility drug Clomid, then months of Clomid with inseminations. During one of our breaks from the treatment, I conceived by accident. What a surprise! We estimated that I was probably three months along. I began bleeding, and within two weeks I miscarried. This was 1989-90. We recovered, and I continued using Clomid for many more cycles until I became severely hyperstimulated and ruptured a huge ovarian cyst. We were told that I should never try Clomid again. I then used Pergonal injections and attempted still more inseminations.

By this time it was 1994. After years of being too scared to attempt GIFT (gamete intrafallopian transfer) or IVF (in vitro fertilization), we took the plunge. We did GIFT using lupron, Pergonal, and metrodin injections, and on our first cycle, I conceived! I soon started bleeding and lost the baby. My doctor did another pregnancy test just to confirm, and to our surprise my hormone level was even higher. Joy turned to despair when we discovered that it was an ectopic pregnancy, which resulted in another laparotomy and the destruction of my one remaining fallopian tube.

After recovering physically and emotionally, IVF was our only option. We did IVF in 1995 using lupron and metrodin. We implanted what we considered a conservative number, four eggs. I was put on bed rest until we found out if I was pregnant. The first pregnancy test showed a level of 1,000 (10 was considered positive), and

I was ordered back to bed until the exact number of babies was determined. I soon began bleeding. It was discovered by ultrasound that I had quadruplets but three were dying, while the baby at the fundus was growing well. I bled constantly and was repeatedly hospitalized. We moved in with my parents so that I wouldn't have to walk down the stairs on my many trips to the emergency room and so that somebody would be near to help take care of me. They rented a hospital bed so that I could be more comfortable.

I had frequent ultrasounds, and at times we couldn't even see the top baby due to the presence of the blood from the other three. I also ruptured an ovarian hemorrhagic cyst and had a 10-centimeter mass behind the uterus. They wanted to do an emergency laparotomy. I was told that saving the one baby was doubtful. I insisted they hold off until the next morning, and by then the mass was miraculously gone.

Throughout the pregnancy I was on complete bed rest with use of a bedside commode or bedpan (my husband is a saint!). I noticed another type of liquid in the bedpan during the times when the bleeding was slow. It proved to be amniotic fluid. They conjectured that the presence of blood in the uterus weakened the amniotic sac around the top baby, causing it to leak for many weeks. I had ultrasounds done every other day, and we discovered that the amniotic fluid index got lower and lower. The sac finally broke, and I lost what little amniotic fluid remained. My body was trying so hard to miscarry. The labor started after the sac finally ruptured. I received magnesium sulfate and was rushed by ambulance to a major university hospital an hour away, with Steve following in hot pursuit.

Because we had tried so hard to get and maintain this pregnancy, the doctors broke medical protocol for us. They gave me magnesium sulfate hoping to ward off delivery even though all amniotic fluid was gone. They normally don't do this because the risk of infection for the mother and baby is so high due to the ruptured sac. I also received steroids. We were told that the baby probably would not survive if it was born within the next two weeks. We were able to hold off delivery for only three agonizing days. Samuel Maxwell Warren was born twenty-one weeks after the IVF (twenty-three weeks after the last menstrual period) in October 1995. We named him Samuel because it means "I have asked God for you" and because, like Hannah, Samuel's mother in the Old Testament, I had previously been unable to conceive.

Early Days, Decisions, and Diagnoses

The decision to use drastic measures to save a much-loved and much-wanted child is probably one of the most difficult decisions anyone could ever make. The doctors told us that they normally wouldn't even try to save a baby so premature, but due to our history of infertility, they would try if we so wished and if it looked as if the baby had a fighting chance. My husband and I agonized over this decision. We desperately wanted this baby we had been trying so hard to have, but we didn't want him imprisioned in a body that wasn't able to function. This is what we told the doctors; it was a wait-and-see decision. When the labor was unstoppable, I delivered my son in a room that was filled with medical personnel from the NICU. I remember the room being very quiet even though there were so many people there. There was no joy or anticipation on anyone's face. My husband and I didn't even get to see our son; he was immediately whisked away, lost from view by the large adult bodies of those trying to save his life.

The entire NICU team was amazed at how big Samuel was. He had always measured large on his ultrasounds, often one or two weeks larger than he really was, thanks to his genes. There was no doubt about his exact age, however, since we knew the precise minute he was conceived in a petri dish! There are many things I love about Steve, but I was never so glad that I married my six-foot-four husband than when they exclaimed about my preemie, "He's huge! He's huge!" Sammy was 1 pound and 8 ounces and 11¾ inches long. Judged in weeks, he should have been less than a pound.

Sammy's Apgar scores were remarkably high (4 and 6), which also surprised everyone. This news was very encouraging and removed all doubt in our minds and the minds of the doctors about saving our baby. We cannot even begin to think of what it would have been like had the original news not been so optimistic.

The positive news and elation soon ended. By the afternoon the doctors were telling us that they didn't expect Sammy to live through the day. They told us that they call the first twenty-four hours after a premature birth the "honeymoon" since the baby remains relatively stable from being inside the mother. Our honeymoon lasted only about five hours; Sammy crashed. The next few months were critical, and he fought for every minute of life. I am still amazed at how fragile and yet strong he was (and still is).

Samuel developed pulmonary interstitial emphysema (PIE), severe bronchopulmonary dysplasia (BPD), pneumothorax (collapsed lung), which required a chest tube, pulmonary edema, two grade II intraventricular hemorrhages (IVH), transient patent ductus arteriosus (PDA), severe anemia and hypoalbuminemia, several severe candidial sepses, which caused his platelets to crash from 300,000 to 6,000, and an inguinal hernia. He also received multiple transfusions of blood and platelets, and a lumbar puncture for suspected meningitis. He was on a high-frequency ventilator and then a traditional ventilator for almost two and a half months. He had terrible bradycardia (dramatic decrease in heartbeat) and apnea (failure to breathe) episodes, often every five minutes. He received IV nutrition called TPN (total parenteral nutrition) for weeks until he was able to tolerate feedings of breast milk by gavage. Once he was off the ventilator we were transferred by ambulance to our local regional medical center for a month-long stay.

Once Sammy was at the medical center, I was able to meet with a wonderful lactation consultant. She let me take Sammy out of the nursery into a private room and helped my husband and me learn how to position Sammy, since he was very small and weak. She would make sure I had plenty of the *four* p's: privacy, pillows, patience, and plenty of towels! Once I took Sam home, she was available to me by phone and would come out once a week to weigh Sammy and help with any problems.

I was very glad that I continued pumping. We didn't find out until five months after his birth that Sammy had an immunodeficiency called hypogammaglobulinemia, which resulted from his severe prematurity. We were so glad that we had been able to give him the immune-rich breast milk even before we found out about his serious immunodeficiency. We both knew how important it was that Sammy continue to receive the immunity from the breast milk, so that kept us going for those twenty-one months. I was able to transition Sammy to nursing, but then he kept getting too sick to nurse and had to be rehospitalized. Finally, after one lengthy hospitalization, he refused to go back on the breast, so I just made the commitment to keep pumping. We are convinced that the breast milk played a key role in keeping him alive and preventing him from getting necrotizing enterocolitis (NEC), a potentially deadly condition in which normally harmless bacteria attack the intestinal wall. This was a powerful motivation for my continuing to pump for so long. The other reason was the incredible support of my husband. From the very beginning he was there with me. We learned together. He never once made me feel weird when I was sitting attached to this machine countless times during the day. He knew that it was something only I could do. He could see what a tiring job it was, so he became my pumping partner and did the round-the-clock schedule with me.

Homecoming

Samuel came home several weeks before his due date, weighing 3½ pounds. He was on continuous-flow oxygen through a nasal cannula. He was hooked up to a monitor that would alarm for any apnea, bradycardia, or tachycardia. He was relatively stable for the first few weeks after coming home but soon became infected with disseminated candidiasis. It started out as diaper rash, but within days it covered the majority of his body and he developed thrush. It spread to the point where it was hard to remember what he looked like without the sores. We were convinced he was near death. He was in so much pain and looked like someone had poured boiling water on him, yet the doctors refused to see him for another office visit for "just" diaper rash and prescribed only very weak topical antifungal medications. I kept telling the doctor that I was sure these sores were an external manifestation of an internal problem. I begged her to hospitalize my son or at least give me a referral for the university hospital where he had been successfully treated before. She finally put Sammy in the local regional center, most probably to get me off her back. This hospital did not have a pediatric ward. They didn't have central A/B monitors so that the nursing station would know when he was bradying. My husband and I did not leave his side for a second because he kept bradying and desaturating. The hospital didn't even have an oxygen flow regulator to measure pediatric levels of oxygen. His face was too broken down to wear the nasal cannula, and it took our insistence and most of the day for them to rig up some sort of an oxygen tent for Sammy.

All they did for him at the hospital was keep his perianal region exposed to air and under a heat lamp to dry the sores. They gave him a mild IV antifungal medicine. When the IV became infiltrated, the doctor was going to send us home on oral medications since there was "nothing more she could do for us." The sores were so bad that they were bleeding, and Sammy was in extreme pain. We missed our beautiful baby: It was so hard to see this bleeding, oozing baby who was reduced to whimpers because he became too weak to scream. We begged her to give him pain medication, but she refused. We begged her to put him on amphotericin due to his history of yeast infections when he was in the NICU. She refused to do this because it would mean transferring him to a tertiary care facility that offered specialized treatment. We insisted that she call in a dermatologist to diagnose the sores, to which she finally agreed. The dermatologist was shocked at what he saw and couldn't believe they weren't putting any strong medicines on the sores to fight the infection. He postulated that it might be a zinc deficiency that was causing the sores.

Only after our desperate pleas for help, our continual demands to be seen by a specialist, and the recommendation from the dermatologist were we finally transferred to a children's hospital where Sammy was put in isolation. We were seen by Pediatric Infectious Disease, Immunology, Hemoncology, and Genetics. They did many blood tests, skin cultures, and a skin punch biopsy. He was diagnosed with a candida infection. At this point we discovered that he had hypogammaglobulinemia; he wasn't making antibodies. The lab result levels were so low that they thought the machine was malfunctioning. He was put on amphotericin yet again to fight the candida. It took nineteen weeks to clear up the infection. They had to surgically place a central thoracic catheter to administer the amphotericin since they couldn't start any more IVs and we had blown two lines for peripherally inserted central catheters. Sammy started to recover due to IV amphotericin, but the thrush and sores still lingered, albeit much improved. We then started using Fungizone, which is a cream form of amphotericin B. Within two days the sores were significantly better; within one week they were almost gone! We also used two treatments of Gentian Violet, which got rid of the thrush.

Due to Sammy's low immunoglobulin levels he was prone to infections and had to be isolated at home. After prolonged and severe respiratory infections through the fall of '96 and the winter of '97, it became necessary to give him gammaglobulin therapy, called IVIG, about once a month. The infusion was given through his central line and lasted about two hours. It caused him significant discomfort. We had to premedicate with diphenhydramine to reduce the reaction and help sedate him.

We continued to keep Samuel isolated at home. We did not give IVIG during the summer months since that is a healthy time of year. Sammy did very well. We retested during the summer of 1997, and his IgA subclasses (antibodies fighting localized infections) were still zero, but his IgG levels (antibodies for past infections) had increased for the first time. We first were ecstatic that he was starting to make his own IgG. However, after both my doctor and I did some research, we realized that we hadn't waited long enough since his last gammaglobulin infusion, and the IgG increase might just be residual from the IVIG, an infusion of antibodies. So we had to keep waiting and praying that he was actually making antibodies.

I returned to work before his first birthday. Samuel received in-home RN care while we were at work because he had to be isolated from others to avoid illness, and had a central thoracic catheter. He was continually sick with upper respiratory infections and ear infections. He required in-home physical therapy twice a week for gross-motor delays. He was also seen once a week by a speech therapist who was a swallowing specialist. She worked with Sammy to help reduce his oral aversion, hypersensitive gag reflex, and swallowing delays.

Sammy was going to turn two in October 1997, and we wanted to have him dedicated at our church. We decided to draw blood levels again right before his second birthday to see what was happening. We found out the Friday before he was dedicated that he was starting to make some IgA for the first time ever, and his IgG was even higher than it was in the summer! Our little one was finally making some antibodies! At first the doctor told us that we could start bringing Sammy out into the world. This was exciting, albeit scary, news. She soon rescinded those orders. Within a week Sammy developed a severe respiratory infection that lasted for the rest of the year. Then he developed a fungal infection on his skin that persisted from the end of December into February 1998. We kept him isolated through April, which coincides with the end of respiratory syncytial virus (RSV) season. We did not give him IVIG but let him fight off the infections without it. We retested his levels in April 1998 and received wonderful news: His IgA had continued to climb, although still below low-normal range, and his IgG also had increased and was now within the low limits of normal! Our prayers had been answered. His central thoracic catheter was not needed anymore, so it was surgically removed. This was even more cause for rejoicing. Our son was now tube free!

Sammy Now

Sammy is now three years old. He is 35 pounds and 38 inches tall. He is still having swallowing problems and is eating stage 3 baby food, but he is making progress and is even feeding himself graham crackers! He has mild speech delays and is amazing us every day by constructing new sentences. He can count to thirty and sing the alphabet. He can recognize and identify all upper- and lowercase letters of the alphabet. He will soon be receiving occupational therapy to address his delays in fine-motor skills.

It has been a very long road living with the fear of infection, having to keep Sammy completely isolated for fear of infection, having to care for his central venous catheter and other medical needs, and trying to provide a stimulating environment for a boy who has never played with another child. Sammy is an outgoing and entertaining boy with a smile that can light up the room. We are enjoying being able to introduce Samuel to the world. Watch out, world, here comes the cutest miracle you've ever seen!

ANNA'S EARLY ARRIVAL

by Craig A. Bright

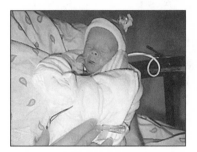

Anna, six weeks old. Mom and Dad visit
the NICU.

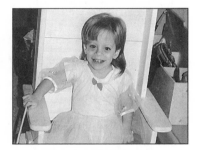

Anna, two years old, dressed for
Halloween.

We had been trying to conceive a child for over two years when my
wife, Kelsey, became pregnant in March 1996. Our efforts to start a
family had included numerous tests and infertility treatments, so
news of the conception brought great joy and relief. About four
months into what had been a routine pregnancy, Kelsey had an unusually high reading on an alpha fetal protein (AFP) test, a screening test that can be an indicator of fetal abnormalities including
birth defects. High levels have also been associated with placental
abnormalities. However, Kelsey had a high-resolution sonogram that
appeared to show a normally developing fetus. When a follow-up
AFP test still came back very high, we opted for an amniocentesis
test as an added precaution. This test, which occurred during the
twenty-first week of gestation, came back normal. In addition,

another sonogram done at the time of the amnio showed the developing baby's size to be on target for the twenty-first week of development. With that good news, we breathed a huge sigh of relief and began to plan for the last trimester.

Kelsey went in for a routine exam five weeks later, on September 11, 1996. Her OB-GYN immediately noticed that Kelsey's abdomen appeared small for twenty-six weeks. He did a quick sonogram in his office and measured the baby's head at twenty-three weeks. At this point he ordered another high-resolution sonogram at a different office. Conducted later that afternoon, this sonogram confirmed the baby's twenty-three-week size. Further, Kelsey's amniotic fluid appeared very low, and the doctor noticed a problem with the blood flow through the umbilical cord. The doctor arranged for us to meet the next day with his colleague, who was a specialist in problem pregnancies and deliveries. Our OB-GYN provided the first sobering assessment that the pregnancy was in serious jeopardy. He noted that a baby delivered at twenty-three weeks of development might not have a very good chance of survival, yet the womb did not appear very hospitable to continued development.

After a horrible night of dread and uncertainty, we met the specialist at 2:30 on Thursday afternoon, September 12. He conducted his own extensive sonogram and confirmed the previous diagnosis of fetal growth reduction, which meant that the baby's growth had not kept pace with normal patterns of development. The doctor noted, however, that the baby did appear to be well formed, and he estimated that just enough amniotic fluid existed to support lung development. He attached a fetal heart monitor to Kelsey. Although the baby's heart rate took several significant dips, it recovered pretty quickly, which the doctor interpreted as a sign of strength. The doctor recommended admitting Kelsey to the hospital, which was adjacent to his office building.

The initial plan involved putting Kelsey on bed rest in the hospital and giving her steroids to build up the baby's lungs so that twenty-four to forty-eight hours later a cesarean section could be performed. Things didn't go as planned. Kelsey was admitted to the hospital around 5:00 P.M. Within half an hour the baby's heart rate took a couple of major dips, causing enough consternation to bring a number of doctors and nurses rushing into the room. After conferring with the specialist, the OB-GYN recommended immediate delivery. He added that "the baby doesn't like it in there anymore" and suggested the baby had a better chance of survival on the outside. Still reeling and basically numb from the events of the past twenty-four hours, we then received a quick five-minute briefing on the course of treatment for premature infants from a neonatologist. She projected that a baby born at twenty-six weeks of gestation but only twenty-three weeks in size had about a 50 percent chance of survival. Compared to our worst fears from the night before, those odds sounded almost reassuring.

The team prepped Kelsey for surgery in about forty-five minutes. Just before the operation, Kelsey indicated through her tears that the baby, known to be a girl, should be named Anna. They wheeled Kelsey into the operating room and gave her an epidural that allowed her to remain conscious. As they pulled her knees up and began to insert the needle, Kelsey looked down at her small belly and thought there was no way someone could get a baby out of there that was big enough to survive. Following the epidural, I went into the operating room and sat with Kelsey. The operation began at 6:30 P.M. At 6:55, the anesthesiologist said, "The baby's been born." I saw Anna briefly just before they wheeled her out to the NICU. Weighing in at 1 pound 5 ounces (585 grams) and not much bigger than the palm of my hand, she looked a little bit like a monkey. Anna's face was tiny, red, and wrinkled. Her arm was the size of a pinky finger. I thought about how unfair it seemed for a child to have to face life outside the protective confines of its mother at such an early stage of development.

After the operation we were so exhausted from the stress of

surgery and the suddenness of the birth that we initially did not think too much about the baby but focused on making sure that Kelsey was okay. We were also afraid that at any minute we might be told that Anna was gone. During a postoperative debriefing with the OB-GYN a short time later, we asked, "How should we view this situation? Should we consider ourselves parents?" He responded, "You are most definitely parents, and no matter what happens you will always be parents."

After enough time had passed for Kelsey to come out of the anesthesia and for the doctors to get Anna stabilized, the nursing staff wheeled Kelsey into the Neonatal Intensive Care Unit (NICU) to see her baby for the first time. Although Anna was hooked up to an array of high-tech monitors and ventilation equipment, we could tell how beautiful she was. We recognized her facial features from the sonograms taken over the past few months. Following this brief visit, we went to a private room on a floor away from the other newborn babies.

I saw Anna about three times during the night while Kelsey tried unsuccessfully to get some much needed sleep. I noted that Anna appeared to be very feisty. Although this was generally viewed as a good sign, the doctors were concerned that given her tiny size and limited reserves Anna might use up too much energy moving around. The next morning she appeared very strong and had passed a very good first night. In part this was the result of Anna's first dose of Surfactant, a medicine developed about a decade ago that can dramatically improve lung performance in premature babies.

Kelsey's father arrived on Friday morning from North Carolina, after driving a good portion of the night, to lend moral support and find out firsthand how his daughter and new granddaughter were doing. Anna's honeymoon period turned out to be disturbingly short-lived. By late in the day on Friday her respiratory performance began to decline and her oxygen requirements increased. After I called from the hospital room to the NICU for an update on Saturday morning, a doctor came in person to speak to us. He indicated that given Anna's deteriorating respiratory condition, she needed to be transferred to a NICU across town that had special ventilators that did less damage to the lungs at high levels of support. The doctor hoped to get Anna's respiration stabilized and then bring her back to the current hospital when her condition improved. Next, a social worker came to talk to us to find out how we were coping. The short answer was: as well as could be expected. The transport team came and got Anna in a spaceship-like incubator at around 10:30 A.M. on Saturday. We watched anxiously as our tiny daughter was wheeled away to face an increasingly uncertain future. The thought of having to deal with an unfamiliar group of doctors and nurses in a large-scale NICU environment at a strange hospital was unsettling.

Kelsey was discharged so that she could visit the baby although less than two days had elapsed since her surgery. It took Kelsey a while to get packed up and checked out, and she had to meet with a lactation specialist about pumping breast milk for Anna. At around 1:30 P.M. we received a call from the new NICU telling us that Anna was gravely ill and in guarded condition, and inquired as to why we had not yet arrived. The doctor added that Anna appeared to have a bacterial infection and high levels of jaundice, and was bleeding in her lungs. We were told that babies who bleed from their lungs typically also bleed into their brains because the tissues are so similar. We were told that Anna needed a complete transfusion (called an exchange transfusion) to replace all her blood, and we were urged to come as soon as possible to sign the required permission forms.

We hailed a cab and headed across town. During the preceding days, several doctors and nurses had told us that we needed to pace ourselves emotionally because the NICU experience was like a roller coaster of good news, bad news, and everything in between. Yet we both were struck by how fast Anna's fortunes had turned from very good to very poor in just a few short hours.

Upon arriving at the NICU, we found Anna in a perilous condition. She required maximum ventilator support as well as manual "bagging" by a nurse to force additional oxygen into her frail and damaged lungs. Not long after, the NICU staff gave Anna the exchange transfusion, started her on a clotting medication to try to stem the lung bleeding, and added a third antibiotic to the two she had already received for her infection. Anna was also placed under bilirubin lights in an effort to reduce her jaundice levels, which were extremely high. She appeared very agitated, and the doctors administered phenobarbital to calm her down. The doctors emphasized that Anna's survival would be an "hour-to-hour" ordeal, with the next twelve hours particularly critical. They were clearly preparing us for the worst and did not want us to have false hope. This focus on the negative, while perhaps necessary, also made our experience even more distressing.

During these earliest stages of the crisis, we were inundated and a bit overwhelmed with inquiries from well-meaning and concerned family members, friends, and coworkers. We found it difficult to manage the flow of information to and from all interested parties, and the drain of hours spent explaining Anna's condition made us feel even more stressed and exhausted. At the same time we found it helpful to talk to others about the experience, and numerous caring souls contributed meals and other acts of generosity that helped ease the burden of getting through the day. Kelsey's mother arrived on Monday to lend additional support.

Several days after Anna's birth, I began sending e-mail updates to my office, Kelsey's office, a few friends, and several family members who had e-mail capabilities. This advancement brought about great efficiencies in communication, significantly cutting the time needed to keep people up to date. The e-mails eventually went out to a list of more than fifty people. They in turn informed many others about Anna's fight for life, and her story touched hundreds of people across the country who said thousands of prayers on her behalf.

Anna managed to hang on through that first difficult weekend. The bleeding in her lungs subsided, and she had enough fight to endure all the complications confronting her. On Monday we received the encouraging news that despite initial suspicions to the contrary, a brain scan showed that Anna had not experienced any bleeding in her head. Later in the day, however, another potential crisis arose when Anna's chest stopped vibrating properly and X rays showed evidence of a "whiteout." The doctors feared a lung hemorrhage or some other type of fluid buildup. It turned out, though, to be a partial collapse of Anna's lung from a reduction in ventilator settings. An adjustment to the machine corrected the problem.

The frequent changes in caregivers complicated our efforts to assess Anna's condition. Anna initially had two nurses tending her for each twelve-hour shift, and different doctors cared for her at different times. We had difficulty figuring out whether an optimistic assessment from a nurse on duty represented real progress or just an upbeat reporting style as compared to other nurses. Conversely, one nurse sent us into a tailspin when she paused and simply responded "Okay" when asked how Anna was doing. In many cases, nurses tended to fall back on statistical recitations in lieu of giving some type of overall assessment. We struggled with the avalanche of medical statistics we received about Anna's condition and tried to figure out how to read them for signs of progress. The numbers included bilirubin counts, blood pressure and heart rate data, red blood cell and platelet counts, ventilator rates and pressures, and oxygen levels and oxygenation percentages. And weight was an ever-present concern. A day could be made or dashed by news that Anna had gained or lost a few milligrams. A nurse who noted our obvious distress over efforts to draw conclusions about Anna's condition told us, "The best thing to do is forget all the numbers and opinions and just concentrate on watching your baby." This was sage advice, given the tendency of parents in the NICU environment to become preoccupied with watching monitors for signs of hope. Over time we became knowledgeable about the peculiarities of Anna's condition and served as an important point of continuity when new caregivers arrived. One nurse, new to Anna, expressed concern about how pale she looked, but Kelsey informed her that was normal for Anna.

As the days following Anna's birth continued to accumulate, we settled into what seemed like a high-stakes waiting game characterized as "bankrolling hours." A doctor told us that the first forty-eight to seventy-two hours after birth were especially critical for babies to get through. Then you start looking at a week for increased chances of survivability, followed by a month. He added that some preemies do die after a month, but not too many. We breathed a little easier when Anna completed day seven.

A few days later we had our first formal conference with Anna's doctors. They reiterated that Anna remained in extremely critical condition but acknowledged that she had made significant progress since her first days. Her bilirubin counts had dropped. Her respiratory performance had improved a bit, but she still required very high levels of breathing support. There was no evidence that the problems facing Anna had done any long-term damage. Those present also acknowledged that Kelsey was doing a great job of religiously pumping breast milk for Anna. The nurses fed Anna the milk in tiny droplets through a feeding tube. The milk made a major contribution to bolstering Anna's primitive immune system.

Day eighteen was memorable for several reasons. Kelsey got to hold Anna for the first time, having yearned to do so since her birth. Tethered to all her tubes and machines, Anna looked a little like an astronaut on a spacewalk outside the protective confines of her incubator. Kelsey marveled at how Anna was so tiny yet perfectly formed, so fragile yet valiant. We agreed that every time we looked at Anna we saw a little glimpse of heaven. The same day the doctors indicated that Anna's respiratory condition had stabilized, and she was ready to return to her birth hospital. We had become comfortable with Anna's care in the NICU, however, and did not want to subject her to any avoidable stresses. When the doctors could not assure us that Anna would not have to return to the NICU in the future, we made the decision to keep her where she was until she could go home.

The next day Anna showed signs of a potential infection. The quick detection by her nurses and prompt administration of antibiotics stopped the problem in its tracks. Things remained relatively quiet until Anna came off the ventilator on October 11, 1996. The next day, a Saturday, Anna had a great one-month birthday party and was breathing well with the support of continuous positive airway pressure (CPAP) nasal tubes that helped keep air pressure in her lungs. Then on Sunday she started having apnea and bradycardia episodes (A's and B's), where her breathing stopped and her heart rate dropped. Sometime during the afternoon she stopped breathing, and the doctors and nurses had to use a manual bagging process to revive her. Apparently a couple of days of breathing on her own had worn out Anna's tiny body, and she had to go back on the ventilator to recharge. It was later determined that Anna also needed a transfusion because her red blood cell count was low, which contributed to her crash. Anna slept for most of the next day just trying to rebuild her depleted reserves. The incident reminded us of the fragility of Anna's condition and emphasized the extent to which we still needed to be ready for anything at any time.

After resting up for about a week, Anna came off the ventilator for good on October 17. The doctors fully weaned her off the CPAP tubes on October 30, at around the seven-week mark. During this time the focus shifted more toward getting Anna to grow. As often occurs with preemies who experience fetal growth reduction, Anna's efforts to gain weight turned out to be an agonizingly slow process. At seven weeks she weighed only 1 pound 13 ounces (810 grams), or a half-pound more than her birth weight. The growth strategy included giving Anna a fat cocktail to supplement the breast milk and keeping her calm to conserve calories.

Around the eighth week we received word that her right eye showed significant signs of retinopathy of prematurity (ROP). Her left eye showed signs of ROP as well but did not appear to be as severely affected. Because ROP carries with it the risk of retinal detachment and blindness, Anna's eye doctors recommended laser surgery to help reduce the chance of permanent visual impairment. They wanted to do the right eye and take a wait-and-see approach with the left eye. Having faced the very real possibility of Anna's death a few weeks earlier, we were relatively unfazed by the risk that she might be blind. The surgery took place in the NICU on November 8. The doctor made sixteen hundred tiny burns around the perimeter of Anna's retina to keep stray blood vessels from growing in toward the center of the eye. Anna received a narcotic for the surgery that left her groggy and brought on numerous A's and B's over the next several hours. We held her for the first couple of hours afterward so we could monitor her vital statistics and shake her awake during each episode. Subsequent exams over the next few months indicated the laser surgery was completely successful. Anna's left eye stabilized and did not require the operation. The doctors warned, however, that like many preemies Anna would likely need glasses at a very early age.

As Anna's condition continued to improve, we were able to hold her for longer and longer periods during daily visits. She began wearing stylish preemie clothes and looking more like a little baby. On November 17, at a little over two months of age, Anna moved to the "step-down" nursery for babies who are not as critically ill. This formal change in Anna's status marked a major symbolic milestone on her road to recovery. On November 19, Anna reached the 1 kilo mark (2 pounds 3 ounces), another important breakthrough. On Friday, December 13, Anna began feeding from a bottle, and the nurses removed her feeding tube. For the first time she had no tubes of any kind going into her body.

Despite these positive indications, the months of daily hospital visits, stress, and waiting for Anna to get big enough to go home continued to drain us. We thought more and more about taking her home and leaving this caring but unnatural environment behind. We handled more and more of Anna's care during visits to the hospital, including changing diapers, taking Anna's temperature, feeding, bathing, and clothing her. She moved to an open crib shortly before Christmas, another prerequisite for going home because it showed Anna could regulate her own body temperature.

Normally the hospital requires babies to reach 4 pounds (1,800 grams) before being discharged. We felt that Anna was being unfairly penalized for being petite, however, and successfully petitioned to have her released at 3 pounds 11 ounces. After we received training in operating Anna's portable heart and breathing monitor and took the required CPR training for infants, we took our little fighter home on January 8, 1998. Anna was 118 days old. My "Annagram" E-mail update for day 118 contained the following excerpts:

> Strangely enough, Kelsey and I weren't nervous about taking Anna home. This was largely because we've had four months to get to know Anna prior to her discharge, and had assumed more and more responsibility for her care at the hospital. And when all was said and done, after all the months of hoping and praying for today, the act of leaving itself was very ordinary. No band played, no fireworks exploded. We wheeled the little one down to the car, strapped her into her car seat, and drove off. And in a way that was the beauty of it. Because if you think back to the times of high drama surrounding Anna's early arrival, one of the

things that kept us going was the simple dream of taking our daughter home just like millions of other parents do every day.

I always imagined we'd fall to our knees and shed tears of joy when we walked in the door. We didn't, because we didn't have time. Your fantasies don't take into account the fact that you have to plug in the monitor, find a pacifier, start mixing up a bottle, prepare to change a diaper, and figure out where exactly to put the little one down.

Anna came home remarkably healthy for the ordeal she had endured. She received four medications, all administered orally. Although she remained hooked up to a portable heart and breathing monitor for a number of months, it never detected any real episodes of A's and B's, and mainly just scared us when its loud, piercing beeps periodically sounded a false alarm. Anna initially had visiting nurses come to the house for a few hours a couple of days a week, but that was quickly discontinued. Weekly appointments with her pediatricians soon gave way to monthly visits. She also received a monthly Respigam vaccine to protect against the dreaded lung virus RSV. This daylong ordeal included an IV that lasted several hours, but the investment helped keep Anna healthy. Although we both got sick at different times, we were careful about rigorous hand washing and sanitation methods, so Anna made it through the winter without catching a cold or flu.

Parents of preemies have a gap between the arrival of their child and the time when they take over from the hospital staff as primary caregivers. We found life at home with Anna to be less stressful than at the hospital but more exhausting. We could no longer leave Anna with the nurses and head home for some rest and relaxation when we got tired. Given Anna's need for someone trained in operating the monitor and administering CPR, and the need to keep Anna isolated to avoid getting sick, we found we had almost no flexibility in taking a break together away from our child care duties. Kelsey also found it increasingly inconvenient and time-consuming to pump breast milk for Anna while taking care of her (Anna never made the transition to breast-feeding), especially since Kelsey had pumped so much more milk than Anna consumed. Although Kelsey stopped pumping around the end of March, she was able to donate a bunch of milk to a milk bank and still have several months' worth left over for Anna.

As several nurses had predicted, once Anna got home she began having crying fits that lasted for several hours each evening. The crying could be mitigated only by walking Anna around in a papoose carrier without stopping. She generally slept through the night, except that we had to get her up every four hours for a bottle to help keep her calorie intake as high as possible. Around February, Anna developed a pretty bad reflux problem that cleared itself up as she grew bigger and adjusted to taking a larger bottle. All of these challenges were greatly overshadowed by the sheer joy that we experienced in caring for a daughter who had barely survived a traumatic birth. As we got to know Anna better and shared more and more of her life, it became harder and harder to recall those early days and think about how close we had come to losing her.

Anna grew dramatically in the months following her homecoming but remains tiny for her age. She weighed 6 pounds in March at six months, 10 pounds at nine months, 14 pounds at fourteen months, and 17 pounds at twenty months in May 1998. But she has never been a great eater, and getting her to down a full meal can be a struggle. Her weight puts her near the bottom of the growth charts, but doctors who thought about growth hormones to help her catch up decided to wait and see what happened. During her second winter Anna experienced numerous ear infections because her ear canals were so small, but she remained generally healthy and had no major setbacks. Although her eyes will require corrective lenses at some point, more recent exams indicate that glasses will not be necessary for a while.

Despite pessimism from developmental experts who warned of possible learning difficulties and developmental delays, Anna has made steady progress on her own deliberate timetable. She began smiling first by accident and then on purpose during February and March 1997. She demonstrated very good hand-eye coordination and was able to grasp objects such as small toys by April. In May she turned over for the first time. The doctors took away her monitor in July. This made us a little nervous, but we made the adjustment. With the help of frequent physical therapy visits, Anna began crawling on her belly by November. Regular crawling on all fours began around Christmas. Anna took her first steps on February 24, 1998, about fourteen months past her original due date, and quickly mastered walking in all its dimensions. Her vocabulary, which consisted of "cat" and "mama" at that time, has slowly but steadily increased.

Today she insistently hands you a book and plops in your lap to hear the story (over and over and over again). She also blows kisses, waves to the moon, points to her nose, ears, and feet, and shows you "how big" she's gotten. She brings you her beach ball if you ask her to, and slides to the floor and dances on demand.

Above all, Anna lives every moment to the fullest. Maybe at some level she appreciates more than most of us how precious and precarious life can be. She has an easy smile and is quick to laugh or shriek with delight. Although Anna is not afraid to unleash a temper tantrum when she doesn't get her way, she loves being around people and is generally eager to please. We try to focus on accepting the blessing of Anna's life without placing too many expectations on her. It is too early to know if Anna will face other developmental obstacles, but we and the many people who have met Anna or know her story would never bet against this stubborn little fighter.

AUSTIN AND ASHLI'S STORY:
THE WORLD OF PREMATURITY

by B. Lynn Shahan

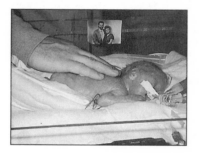

Ashli, three weeks old.

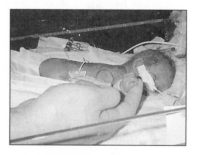

Austin, three weeks old.

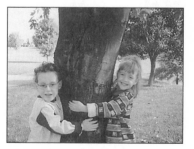

Austin and Ashli, four years old.

Our story begins in November 1994. I was on my way home from work and was coming down with a cold, so I stopped at our local drugstore to get some medication. On my way to the drug counter I thought to myself, "Better make sure we're not having a baby before

I dope myself up on medicine." That was a good idea, for I took the pregnancy test and *whammo!* It was positive. Later that week David and I were chatting about how far along I was. We pinpointed it around four weeks. I said to him, "That check mark on the pregnancy test showed up fast. Do you think it could be twins?" He said, "No. Two check marks would have appeared if that was so!"

After Christmas I called my obstetrician because I was having serious pain in the lower part of my stomach. A complete physical exam could not find any reason for the pain. The doctor suggested an ultrasound to investigate further. At the beginning of the ultrasound my husband asked the doctor, "Just what are the odds of us having twins?" He told the doctor there was a history of twins in our family. The doctor said, "This is your first pregnancy, and most twin pregnancies are flukes and often do not occur in a first-time pregnancy." The assistant doing the ultrasound spoke up and said, "Take that all back. The reason she's in pain so early is there are two!" My husband's eyes got really big, and he sank to the floor. At seven and a half weeks, we knew we were having twins.

Victims of Preterm Labor

For the first four months it seems I had all-day sickness, not morning sickness. This was very hard on me because I worked full-time as an administrative assistant in a state office. I was finally okayed for a reduced workweek, which allowed me to have Wednesdays to build up energy. (I still say if I hadn't pushed this, I would not have carried Austin and Ashli as long as I did.) Once the all-day sickness began to cease, I had just a few weeks of "the norm."

On April 8, 1994, I phoned my OB about a severe pain in my back. Earlier I had been told my stomach was already so tight I would only feel contractions in my back. My OB instructed me to go to the emergency room. They checked out my complaint and found I was 1 centimeter dilated. They kept me for a twenty-four-hour observation, put me on medications, and gave me a shot that would stop the preterm contractions. On April 9 they had me walk around periodically for a couple of hours. They gave me another exam and concluded the dilation had stopped. I was to go home, have complete bed rest, and take Brethene, a medication to stop labor, at the onset of contractions (or, in my case, when severe back pain set in).

This was effective for a week. I went in on Thursday, April 14, 1994, at 4 P.M. My OB found I was 4 centimeters dilated and panicked. He basically said we had to stop this immediately. My husband was instructed to take me via wheelchair to the Labor and Delivery Hall while my OB made some phone calls. Hindsight now tells me he was informing the NICU. During the hectic process of being put in a delivery room, a nurse came in and examined me. She ran into the hall and yelled, "She's a nine. Get her OB here *stat!*" We did not know what "she's a nine" meant. She came back and immediately gave me what I thought was a shot. I said, "Oh, that's that miracle stuff. It will stop these contractions." The nurse looked at me, at my husband, and then back at me, and said, "Honey, you're nine centimeters dilated. We can't stop a thing. You're having these babies *now!*" We could do nothing but cry.

The Premature Delivery

From the moment the nurse said, "You're having these babies now," it seems we were pulled into the climax of a movie. There must have been twenty-five or more people in the delivery room. I was approached by a gentle-looking man who informed me he was the head of the Neonatal Intensive Care Team for the hospital and that he would be taking over the care of my babies from birth. Little did I know that this man would play one of the biggest roles in my life: saving my children. He asked my husband to step aside for further conversation; I did not have a clue what they were talking about, but I could see my husband beginning to cry. I began to cry more. Were my babies going to be born dead? They returned to my side, and the neonatologist spoke softly. "I told your husband that if the babies attempt to breathe, they will have the strength to do it for only a very short while. Your husband has told us to assist. Do you agree?" I looked at David, then back at the man, and sobbed, "Yes, save my babies."

Within the next twenty-five minutes my twins were born. At 5:06 P.M. came Austin Michael Shahan; he weighed 1 pound 8 ounces and was 13 inches long. At 5:13 P.M. came Ashli Marie Shahan; she weighed 1 pound 4 ounces and was 12.25 inches long. They were intubated immediately after birth and bagged with 100 percent oxygen, among many other routine medical procedures. They were then transported down the hall to the Neonatal Intensive Care Unit (NICU). This would be our home for the next four months.

My First Impression

It was almost midnight when I awoke, startled. I thought to myself, "I am sleeping on my stomach. That can't be. I'm pregnant with twins." Slowly, partial reality came to me. I was in a hospital room and no longer pregnant. Next, I found myself wandering the hall; my husband woke and followed me. "Where are my babies?" I sobbed. A kind nurse sat me down and began to explain it all to me again, as if it were the first time. My babies had been born at 5:06 P.M. that evening, at twenty-four weeks and five days' gestation. As it all came back to me, I began to cry even harder, remembering the tiny bodies I had seen earlier. Until now it had all seemed like a terrible nightmare, but it was real. The nurse said to my husband and me, "Go see your babies. Right now you need them as much as they need you."

A journey through some double doors led us to the NICU, whose doctors and nurses would become extended family. Nothing can prepare you for the overwhelming effects of the NICU. It is a world of its own, one that you do not know exists unless your life takes you there. That first night I looked at all the machines and followed all the wires and tubes that led to my tiny babies. I zeroed in on their belly buttons, where tubes and lines were entering their bodies—the works of a "mechanical mommy" filling in where my body had left off. This was a good thing, I told myself, and at that point the intimidation of it all began to cease.

We remained with our little ones until 3 A.M. The atmosphere of the NICU is horrible, and I would not wish anyone the experience. But today, as I look at my twins, Austin and Ashli, I continue to thank God. My husband and I gave the twins life, but it is He and the knowledge and skill of the NICU that allow them to be with us now.

Roller-Coaster Ride

On April 14, 1994, my husband and I (along with close family members) got on what seemed to be a never-ending roller-coaster ride. This coaster was going full steam ahead, and the constant ups and downs were enough to just blow you away! As David and I look back on it now, we have absolutely no idea how we got through the next four months, the next year, this past year, and so on. Our only explanation is that we had each other and the power of God behind us.

After a few days in the hospital, I was released to go home without my babies. Oh, how I hated to leave them behind, but we had no choice. My days would now be made up of:

- getting up in the morning
- pumping my breasts
- getting dressed
- eating whatever I could tolerate due to my nerves
- answering and making a million and one phone calls
- pumping my breasts again
- finally leaving for the hospital
- loving and nurturing my twins to the best of my ability

- meeting my husband there in the early afternoon
- eating dinner in the hospital cafeteria
- spending the rest of the evening with the twins
- returning home and pumping my breasts again
- phoning the NICU between 11 p.m. and 12 a.m. to check on the twins
- going to sleep in order to get up and start all over again

Each new day brought different ups and downs on the coaster. One day Ashli would do well and Austin not so well; the next day it would be the opposite. Rarely did we receive a good report on both twins on the same day. And just when we got confident that one of them was doing fine, he or she would prove us wrong. By the end of Austin and Ashli's first week of life, our coaster began to take a nosedive.

Austin's Fight for Life

On April 21, at seven days old, Austin had to have life-saving surgery. This is how it began: My husband, David, was on his way back to work for the first time since the twins were born. We called the NICU very early that morning to see how the twins were doing. We noticed some nervous answers when it came to Austin. They basically told us that his stomach had started to swell during the night, the neonatologists were watching him closely, but nothing had been determined yet. David, feeling as though he had no choice, left for work.

At around 8:30 a.m. the neonatologist phoned personally; I knew this was serious. He informed me that Austin would be going in to surgery immediately and for me to get there as soon as possible. I even had to give them consent over the phone in case I did not get there in time. I phoned David, then ran next door and asked for a ride, but David was able to come back for me so we could go to the hospital together.

By 9:30 A.M. the NICU waiting room was filled with David and me, our pastor, and my mother and father, all anxiously waiting to hear from the surgeons. A neonatologist had informed us that Austin was suffering from necrotizing enterocolitis (NEC) that resulted in a perforated bowel. For any premature baby this was a serious condition. The surgeon finally came to say, "Pray and cross your fingers. He is so few days of age and so low in weight, his strength to pull through will be limited. Go spend a few minutes with Austin." This told us Austin's chances were slim.

Crying now seemed to have no end. A sea of tears had been shed since April 14, and now there were to be more. We all gathered around and began to pray while taking turns to be with Austin. I was the last to see him. While at his side, my words were the last for him to hear:

Austin, my dear, sweet, tiny boy, YOU PROVE THEM WRONG. Honey, you fight! Austin, if you pull through, I, your mommy, will dedicate my life to you and your sister and any other family that is drawn into this world of prematurity. Please, Austin, draw your strength from me and all the others praying for you! Fight, Austin, fight!

Soon after I spoke these words they began the process of taking my dear, sweet, tiny boy to surgery. Everybody gathered in the hall to watch him go, and for the next two hours we were in the waiting room.

A Mother's Tears

David and I held each other, crying and fearing the loss of our son. Our hearts were his. I continued praying and sending him the message, "Fight, Austin, fight." While our pastor talked and prayed with us, I prayed, "Lord, let it be your will that he makes it through the surgery." I also asked for a sign: "I am putting it in your hands, Lord, but please give me a sign."

I looked down at the arm of the chair. It had four teardrops on it. One tear had smeared just a little. I was in somewhat of a trance, but I immediately focused on the face that these teardrops had formed: two eyes, a nose, and a mouth. The face of my son. I thought, "This is my sign. As long as I continue to look at this face, I will be able to feel his presence and the life that remains in him." The tears faded away, but I fully believe it did not happen until the surgery was over and Austin made it through.

Ashli's Next Three Months

Austin came through the surgery and stayed in critical condition for a couple of weeks. While he was recovering from his first surgery, darling little Ashli seemed to be having smaller ups and downs. Think of how a tiny kitten is born with its eyes still fused together. Well, Ashli's were also. She began to open them around day eleven of her life. During her first week we had a scare with her also: Her bilirubin began to soar. When it reached a count of twelve, the only choice was a complete blood exchange. Fortunately, they were able to conduct the exchange at her bedside, so we could be with her.

We were told that little girl preemies do better than little boy preemies, and Ashli and Austin were model examples of this. After her blood exchange, she tackled all the "normal" micropreemie problems, such as getting off the ventilator, working toward getting off oxygen (which she didn't succeed at until she came home), and being treated for sepsis. Then during her second month she accompanied Austin in surgery for retinopathy of prematurity (ROP). This was laser surgery to help keep her retina from detaching and eventually causing her to go blind. She was removed from the ventilator and never returned to it (except a short while during the ROP surgery). She made her way from an oxygen hood to a nasal cannula within a few weeks. For the next month, June 15 to July 15, she became an eater and a grower. She went through the IV feedings, continuous tube feedings through the nose, and bolis feedings (measured feeding through the nose but not continuous). This was used to adapt her to scheduled feedings. Then finally we got to nippling! We had a time with her when it came to eating. If she choked, she wouldn't cough and revive herself. She would just shut down. Her alarms would go off and scare us something awful. We dealt with this for three more months before she got the hang of nippling without choking.

On July 15, 1994, before her due date of August 1, Ashli was released from the NICU at a whopping 4 pounds 7 ounces. While getting her dressed in a darling preemie outfit to take home, across from her was our Austin dealing with yet another mountain to climb.

Austin's Next Four Months

Austin had survived his first surgery, a big fight for a baby so small and so sick. After the ileostomy was created, he remained in critical condition for two weeks. The biggest scare was infection while his internal wounds were healing. His little body was so swollen, he appeared to have gained weight, which actually made him look good. We were told by the nurses not to be deceived by his appearance. Once the swelling went down he would be back to his 1½-pound weight.

Austin slowly began to take on a normal course of treatment, similar to Ashli's. But at six weeks Ashli had already weaned herself from the ventilator. For Austin the medication Indocin did not work to close his patent ductus arteriosus (PDA). This valve in the heart should close at birth, but it often does not happen in preemies. He had been given one round of Indocin prior to his bowel perforation, then two more rounds after the recovery from his first surgery. Because of the delay with the last two Indocin treatments, the proper results did not occur—the spontaneous closing of the PDA on its own. So in May little Austin went in for his second surgery, a type that was routinely done before the invention of Indocin. The surgeon physically clamped the heart valve shut. Austin came out of this surgery again in critical condition.

As the weeks passed, he again took on a normal course of treatment similar to Ashli's. In June, Austin and Ashli both went in for the laser surgery on both eyes. In July, when Ashli was coming home, we brought Austin a cute outfit and dressed him up as if he were going home, too, but he wasn't. Our little boy's future was again on hold. Since the ileostomy was created during his first surgery, feedings were not easy for him. Tolerating any type of feeding other than IV feedings was not possible. He seemed to be fading away. He developed rickets (brittle bones) from a vitamin D deficiency. His little body was discolored from the continuous IV fluid, and he was not gaining weight. The head neonatologist of Austin's care and his former surgeon decided it was time to reconnect Austin's intestines and close the ileostomy. On August 3 this would be Austin's fourth surgery while in the NICU. Each time he left us to go into surgery, it got harder and harder. This time we held on to the thought that this would be his last, the one that would allow him to come home and be with his mommy, daddy, and twin sister. Austin came out of this surgery again in critical condition, but once he had a few days to begin recovering, it was as if he also knew this surgery was needed in order to go home! The neonatologists had predicted we would not have him home until sometime in September, but Austin had other plans. As soon as he had recovered enough to start feedings, we started him on breast milk, and he ate and ate and ate! He tolerated every increase in feedings and began to gain weight immediately. Amazingly, we were able to take him home on August 11, 1994, weighing a whopping 4 pounds 12 ounces! Our family of four was together at last!

Austin and Ashli Then

By the time Austin came home, Ashli was used to her home. Before, when both were in the NICU, we could visit them together. We could take turns with them and feel we were giving them equal amounts of attention. But with Ashli at home and Austin in the NICU, Mom and Dad became torn between the happy, healthy, growing little girl at home and their little boy still in the NICU, not eating, not thriving, and in desperate need of surgery. I still feel this was one of the hardest times we had to endure.

On the evening of August 11, 1994, we left the hospital for the last time. The roller coaster we had begun to ride on April 14, 1994, at ninety-nine miles per hour was now slowing down. Would it come to a complete stop anytime soon? This was now the big question. Our small home became a mixture of routine and chaos. Sounds redundant, right? Well, not with a set of preemie twins. Not only did we have the normal things you do with a newborn times two, but also all the preemie-related things to do times two. We quickly discovered that in the middle of chaos there had to be routine. A day for us included:

- feedings every three to four hours times two
- rocking and putting to sleep every three to four hours times two
- medicines every three to four hours times two
- changing diapers as needed times two
- nebulizer treatments every four hours times two
- pumping my breasts every four hours
- washing and scalding bottles twice daily
- washing their laundry
- keeping individual records consisting of *everything* we did on a daily basis
- routine home health care visits by a nurse every three or four days

And these are just the things that, four years later, I can remember vividly. It seemed every hour of the day it was time for something! We managed somehow on few meals, little sleep, and maybe a shower here and there. This was our life; the roller coaster had not stopped. But I can say we did live through it.

Things seemed to go well until two things happened. The twins were weaned from breast milk to formula, and the winter months arrived. In October 1994 I had played super mom to the fullest extent, and something had to give. It was so hard for me to give up the one thing I had been doing for my babies from day one—pumping my breasts for their milk. It became my rock, my sanity in this whole experience, and to give it up was a painful decision to make. But I did for my well-being and for that of the rest of the family. To attest to the importance of breast milk for preemies, once the twins went to straight formula at the end of December, they immediately became sick. We battled sickness until the spring of 1995. Fortunately, neither twin had to be rehospitalized during that winter. We feel what saved us was total isolation; we remained under what we called house arrest all winter.

During those months we did have visits from the required nurses and from one other program, Early Intervention (E.I.). This program also became a part of our lives. E.I. concentrates on the idea that children at risk need intervention early to help them later in life. E.I. has done so many wonderful things for us. For example, I am an only child and never did a lot of baby-sitting as a teenager. I knew nothing about the development of a normal newborn baby, infant, or toddler, let alone babies that were going to be late in development. So I am very grateful that E.I. taught me what children should be doing at each stage in development. On Austin and Ashli's first birthday, E.I.'s family coordinator brought them two presents: a set of stacking cups and a shape-sorter bucket. She told me before she left, "Now don't put those toys away thinking they are not old enough for them yet. Put them with the rest of their toys and let them do what they want with them—even if it isn't what they are supposed to." I did just that. They explored them at their own pace and in no time were trying to stack and sort them. This became a rule in our house. We did not buy all age-appropriate toys but bought developmental toys that were just a little too old for them. This has worked wonders in helping them become age-appropriate. By April 14, 1995, Austin and Ashli seemed to be coming along all right. Their delays were within the realm of their adjusted age and actual age.

During 1995 we started to see that Austin and Ashli were going to be two totally different individuals, developing at a completely different pace. Austin crawled in April 1995. Ashli did not crawl until June. Austin walked in July, and Ashli walked in late December. Ashli was struggling more with BPD and was hospitalized for lack of oxygen during the winter. We slowly came to realize that even though Austin had the rougher beginning, Ashli might have more long-term effects of her prematurity. By April 14, 1996, when Austin and Ashli were two years old, they seemed to be the equivalent of fifteen- to eighteen-month-olds. From that point on they seemed to keep a delay of around six to nine months. Minor cognitive and developmental delays were becoming more noticeable, but we really began to notice the prevalence of strong speech delays in both of them. It also was clear that potty training was nowhere in the near future. Yet we seemed to sail through the terrible twos, and this fooled us. We thought we had been given a break due to all we had been through! *Not!*

Three and Four Years Old

By April 1997 when Austin and Ashli were three years old, they decided to participate in the terrible twos, so we renamed them the terrible threes. This was the year we said good-bye to Early Intervention. During the last two years the twins had received speech therapy and physical therapy, and had attended play groups to help them with developmental delays. At this time, speech seemed to be their biggest delay. At three their speech was the equivalent of a two-year-old. Leaving E.I. meant venturing into another world of special services. The twins tested eligible for services through the Board of Education. This meant the board would follow their needs through to kindergarten and beyond if needed. It was decided by a team that the best way to meet Austin's and Ashli's needs would be for them to be around other typically developing same-aged children. So it was set that on September 5, 1997, they would both start a Head Start preschool program. They would have a special education teacher work with them set hours a week along with their Head Start teacher. Also, a speech therapist would come twice a week to work with them on their speech delays. I really wondered how Austin and Ashli would adjust to this weekly routine of four half days of school because they had been isolated so much for most of their lives. And to *want* to go to preschool on a daily basis seemed to be asking too much. But Austin and Ashli proved us wrong. I stayed with them for two weeks and then began a phase-out period. I think it was harder on me than on them. Preschool was a hit! They were slow to make friends and actually play with other children, but this was expected. During their first year of preschool, they grew and changed a great deal in knowledge, personality, and character. I came to see that our goal of their starting kindergarten on time was not out of reach.

In the summer of 1998, Austin and Ashli seemed like typical four-year-olds. Austin finally had to get glasses, which had been anticipated for over a year, but his pediatric ophthalmologist was not able to determine if his need for glasses was entirely related to his retinopathy of prematurity. He got little gold-rimmed glasses with little colored trains on either side. He seemed to take to them fairly well, and only time will tell if we will conquer yet another battle—with a lazy eye. Ashli still has BPD, but in the winter she was not hospitalized for oxygen, a sign that she may be outgrowing it. But for now she is diagnosed with seasonal childhood asthma. Austin and Ashli still have speech delays, but they seem to be diminishing. And, finally, we can travel without taking diapers with us. For the most part, they are completely potty trained. They are still small in size and weight, around 28 pounds and 37 inches tall. At four they are fortunate to have few permanent reminders of their beginning. When they were released from a high-risk clinic a year ago, a neonatologist said to us, "To have one micropreemie do this well is a miracle. But to have two, I have no explanation. You simply beat the odds twice."

Looking Back

I look back on how they had to fight to be where they are today, and tears form in my eyes every time. In 1994, Austin and Ashli were born fifteen weeks before their time. They conquered every statistic. Each time they were expected to have a setback, they leaped forward. I still remember our neonatologist saying to us within the first two days of birth, "These little babies know only how to fight. Giving up is a learned process that, fortunately, they have not been taught yet!" And our twins must have heard him say that because at four years old their prematurity has left few lasting effects on them. As for their parents, the fact that Austin and Ashli were born so prematurely will *never* leave us completely. The tiny scars on their feet and hands are just one daily reminder of their early beginnings. As for the roller-coaster ride we took in 1994, we have gotten off. I smile and think to myself, "We got off the prematurity roller coaster just in time to take the roller coaster of life." I am so thankful we can do just that. I will end Austin and Ashli's story with our own personal quote: "Prematurity is a world you never know exists unless life takes you there."

BO: MY MIRACLE BABY

by Cori Layne Smith

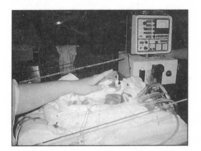

Bo, one week old.

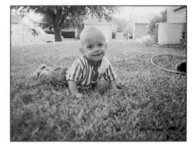

Bo, one year old.

I'm the mother of two wonderful boys. My first son, Jake, was born one month early, at thirty-six weeks' gestation, due to preeclampsia. I was very young and scared. Jake was born weighing 6 pounds 7 ounces and was able to come home with me right away. Seven years later I attempted to have another child. I had remarried, and my husband and I had one son each; we wanted them to have another sibling. I became pregnant almost instantly. We kept an eye on my blood pressure, but everything looked good. At about eight weeks into the pregnancy I went in for a regular sonogram, and it was determined that I had miscarried at about the fourth or fifth week. I was heartbroken but vowed to keep trying.

Three months later I became pregnant again. This time I was scared to death and didn't tell anyone (friends or coworkers) until I hit the "magic" time of three months. I was very excited and was eagerly anticipating the arrival of my second child. At some point all the signs of pregnancy disappeared. Panicked, I ran into my OB's office, husband in tow. I did not want to face this loss alone. A vaginal ultrasound showed again that my baby had died somewhere in the eighth to tenth week. My husband and I both sat in the exam room and cried. They offered to let me miscarry naturally or do a D & C. We chose the D & C because I didn't want to sit home and cry while waiting for my traitorous body to expel this greatly wanted child.

After the D & C I was told to wait about three months before trying again. I wanted my doctor to run tests and find out why my body could not carry a baby. He kept telling me that after three miscarriages we would have reason to justify infertility tests. I was furious but decided to try again. I was diagnosed as a "habitual aborter."

About three months later I became pregnant again. I didn't even tell my husband for fear of losing this one, too. It was during Christmas, and we were around my cousin who had a beautiful baby girl. It was so hard to be near her and not cry my eyes out for what I had lost. While we were at my aunt's home, I began bleeding again. I was probably only four or six weeks along, but it still hurt. I went to my OB's office armed with all sorts of articles from the Internet about different reasons for miscarriages. He was very open to reading and discussing them, and we agreed to go ahead with the testing.

The first test was a hysterosalpingogram (HSG). It is essentially an X-ray procedure in which a radio-opaque dye is injected through the cervix into the uterus and fallopian tubes. This dye appears white on the X ray and allows the radiologist and doctor to see if there are any abnormalities, such as an unusually shaped uterus, tumors, scar tissue, or blockages in the fallopian tubes. This test showed no abnormalities, so we moved on to the next test. On a positive note regarding the HSG, it has been proven that the dye somehow makes the uterus more susceptible to allowing an egg to attach to the uterine wall. I held on to this information with a ray of hope although my problem had been maintaining a pregnancy, not conceiving.

The next test was an endometrial biopsy. This procedure involves scraping a small amount of tissue from the endometrium shortly before menstruation is due. The test is used to determine if a woman has a luteal phase defect, a hormonal imbalance that prevents a woman from sustaining a pregnancy because not enough progesterone is produced. This test showed that my body was *not* producing enough progesterone. Finally, we were getting somewhere.

Next we did some blood tests to see if I had an autoimmune disorder. An autoimmune disorder can cause the rejection of a pregnancy and means the woman is rejecting her own proteins; in other words, she is treating them like an invading illness. I was tested for antiphospholipid antibodies (APA) and lupuslike anticoagulants. Both came up positive. The APA antibodies themselves do not cause miscarriage, but their presence indicates that an abnormal autoimmune process will likely interrupt the ability of the phospholipids to do their job, putting a woman at risk for miscarriage, second trimester loss, intrauterine growth retardation (IUGR), and pre-eclampsia. About 4 percent of women with recurrent miscarriage test positive for lupuslike anticoagulant (LAC), which I did. Women with the LAC antibody are at high risk for implantation failure due to the blood's clotting too fast. When this occurs, the pregnancy is interrupted by a spontaneous abortion, usually during the first four months.

Now that I knew what I was facing, my doctor and I devised a plan. I was to start immediately on baby aspirin to thin my blood. Once I conceived, I was to begin taking prednisone, a steroid that acts as an immunosuppressant. Aspirin therapy, sometimes in concert with prednisone in severe cases, can increase blood flow to the placenta by inhibiting the tendency for clotting in women with abnormal levels of autoantibodies. He also prescribed progesterone suppositories to increase my hormone levels to those needed to sustain a pregnancy.

In February 1997 I conceived Bo, my miracle baby. By this time I knew what I needed to do to achieve a successful pregnancy and began the drug therapy. I took the medications religiously and prayed that these would get me through this last chance of a normal pregnancy. The pregnancy progressed smoothly. I gained an outrageous amount of weight due to the steroids, but I was okay with this because I would get a baby from it. Because of all the previous miscarriages, I was monitored very closely and had sonograms done on a regular basis. During one of the many ultrasounds, we found out that I was carrying a boy, and we decided to name him Bo Robert Smith.

At fifteen weeks, while at work, I began to bleed. I rushed home in a panic, thinking I was miscarrying. My doctor's office told me to come in immediately. When my husband and I arrived, we were escorted to the sonogram room. We were both terrified of what we would see. I was crying and praying and hoping against hope that everything would be okay. The doctor did a vaginal sonogram and then promptly removed it, stating that it looked as if I had placenta previa. An external ultrasound confirmed the placenta previa and, more important, that the baby was fine. In placenta previa the ovum implants on the weaker lower portion of the womb, causing the placenta to grow over all or part of the cervical canal. As the placenta grows and becomes heavier, the weaker portion of the uterus is not able to give sufficient support. The placenta may stretch and thin out, and may tear and begin to bleed. Painless bleeding in either the second or third trimester is the only symptom of this potentially life-threatening situation for both mother and baby.

At this point I was admitted to the hospital until the bleeding stopped or slowed down. I spent eight days in the hospital in bed, getting up only to use the bathroom. During this time I missed my first son's seventh birthday party. I cried the whole day and even when they came to see me after his party and brought pictures. I was so depressed and scared. My husband insisted on staying with me every night because he was afraid I would die and he wouldn't be there. This was such a stressful time for all of us. My son stayed with my mother, and my husband's son, Cy, went to stay with his mother in Oklahoma.

In the hospital I was taken off the prednisone, progesterone, and baby aspirin. I remember hating to go to the bathroom because I was afraid of what I might find. The bleeding began to taper off, and I was allowed to go home. My instructions were to stay off my feet. The bleeding was still present but had turned to "old" blood and looked as if it would stop at any time. For nine weeks I stayed home and worried. I still saw my doctor regularly, and during one appointment after an ultrasound I was told that the previa had moved up. I was excited at this news but a little surprised since I still had spotting. It was determined after another look at the ultrasound that I had a blood clot sitting on the top of my cervix. Since this wasn't as serious as the previa, we were all able to relax a little. My bed rest was modified, and I was allowed to take my sons to football practice and be a spectator. I felt as though I had won the lottery. I wasn't used to this much freedom! I was finally starting to show and went out and bought all kinds of cute maternity clothes.

On August 12, my twenty-ninth birthday, I had lunch with some dear friends from work to celebrate. I ate like a horse, and they enjoyed my looking pregnant. When I had left work to begin the bed rest, I hadn't been showing at all, so they got a big kick out of it. That afternoon, while watching television, it felt as if my period had started. Once again I had started to bleed. It wasn't bad, but it was fresh blood, which scared me to death! I immediately called my OB, and we rushed to the hospital. Another ultrasound showed that the baby was okay. My doctor said it was probably just leftover blood from the previa, but just in case, I was admitted for monitoring. I was hooked up to a fetal monitor and blood pressure monitor in a labor and delivery room. Bo was still so small that they had trouble keeping track of him in the womb. The nurses would get a good reading of his heartbeat, and then he'd go swimming off. It was quite comical, and I was relaxed because I didn't sense any imminent danger. My husband had gone home to get the boys, and we all sat in the room together. My seven-year-old absolutely refused to leave my side. He kept watching the fetal monitor print out and listening to Bo's heartbeat. Finally the bleeding stopped and everything looked fine, so I was able to return home.

That night was uneventful, but the next night was another story. Another trip to the bathroom had worse results. I was bleeding again, so I contacted the doctor on call since it was after hours. He told me to come in, but I talked him out of it because I was sure it was just going to be a replay of the previous night. I promised to come in if the bleeding got any worse. I propped myself on the couch, feet up, and tried to relax. The next thing I knew, I had a gushing feeling. I was bleeding so badly that I was passing large clots of blood. This all began at about 10:30 at night, so both boys were asleep.

My husband rushed me to the hospital after waking Cy, who is fourteen, and telling him we were leaving. They had school the next day, so we didn't want to drag them out again. We got to the ER, and we were sent to a room up on the labor and delivery floor again. The admitting person asked if I wanted a wheelchair, but I said I could walk. I was still thinking it was just a replay of the previous night, so my husband and I were joking and laughing on the way up. By the time we got to the room, my pants were soaked with blood, and then I started to panic. The nurse hooked me up to all the monitors and had me lie on my left side. My blood pressure was through the roof at this time, and they were getting concerned. I was just in for monitoring, so the doctor didn't even stop by. As I lay there in the hospital bed, I kept feeling gushes of blood. No matter what I did, it wouldn't stop.

Finally, I insisted that the nurse page the doctor. He showed up about thirty minutes later and started explaining what was going to happen. He brought in a sonogram machine and verified that Bo was still doing okay. He said the bleeding was not slowing down, so he wanted to transfer me to a hospital with a level III NICU just in case. I kept telling him that I would stop bleeding and everything would be okay, but if it made *him* feel better to transfer me, then okay. (I had never met this doctor before even though he was in the same practice with my doctor, so I was a little concerned.) The doctor asked what I wanted done if he had to deliver Bo. I wasn't sure what he meant, but if he was asking if I wanted him to save my baby, then, yes, he should do whatever was necessary. I was shocked that he had to ask, and he explained that some parents choose not to resuscitate and let nature takes its course. I was still positive that this would not end with my delivering at twenty-four weeks, so I wasn't too concerned. He said he had called my doctor, who was planning to meet us at the other hospital. I asked him to explain to my husband what was going on because I just couldn't think clearly or speak anymore. So we woke my husband up and explained what was happening.

By the time I arrived at the other hospital by ambulance, it was about three or four in the morning. I was rushed to an OB-GYN critical care room. Seeing that sign made me realize I was in real trouble. They began hooking me up to all the monitors again and were having trouble finding little Bo. The doctor came in, found him right away, and did another ultrasound. Everything looked okay except for the heavy bleeding. At this point my husband and I decided to call my mother, and she and my stepfather rushed over to the hospital immediately. They had just come into my room when Bo's heart rate slowed dramatically. The nurse said it was probably due to his flipping around and tangling in the umbilical cord. I relaxed a little and started explaining to my mom and stepfather what was happening. The nurse turned the monitor down so that I couldn't hear it anymore, calmly tore off the sheet with the heart rate readout, and then left the room. I was certain the bleeding would soon stop and figured I would have to stay until it did.

Imagine my surprise, shock, and terror when the doctor came bursting into the room with a group of people wearing surgery masks and caps. He told me that Bo was in distress and they had to take him now. The anesthesiologist came at me with an epidural needle and told me to bend over. I started arguing that I wasn't in labor, and he said, "You're fixing to be!" All my family was taken out of the room, and I was prepped for an emergency cesarean section. I was crying and shaking uncontrollably, and the nurses kept telling me that I needed to calm down. I have never been as terrified in my whole life as I was at that moment.

In the middle of all this, I kept asking the doctor, "Why, why, why?" He told me we had to do this to save me and the baby. As I was being wheeled down the hall to the operating room, I looked at my family; they were all petrified but trying to put up a brave front for me.

I found out later that my placenta had abrupted. A placental abruption occurs when the placenta begins to deteriorate and prematurely separate from the uterine wall. Depending on the stage of the pregnancy and the severity of the separation, the fetus could be deprived of oxygen and essential nutrients, leading to premature labor and even fetal death. As with placenta previa, the mother is at risk of internal bleeding and hemorrhaging.

When I arrived in the OR, a mass of people was rushing around in what seemed like a panic. I was crying and shaking and looking around to see what was going on. A man with a mask, who I later found out was the neonatologist, introduced himself and told me that he would take care of my baby. I kept asking if my baby would be okay, knowing that the chances were not good. They placed the sheet at about my breastbone, and I really started to freak. I wanted to prevent this from happening, so I started arguing with the doctors, saying that I still had feeling in my legs and please don't cut yet.

I was terrified beyond belief, and then an angel, a wonderful nurse, sat beside me and took my hand. She told me that she was the mother of a twenty-four-weeker, too, and he was now almost sixteen and "fixin' to drive." Hearing that made me feel so much better. It seemed like a ray of hope, and I grabbed on and held fast. As she sat there and tried to calm me, she told me that my husband would sit with me. I told her there had to be a mistake because he had told me that he wouldn't be in the room when the baby was born. This had been a pretty big argument throughout the pregnancy. He came and sat down and took my hand. When I looked into his eyes, all I could see was love, compassion, and, of course, terror. I kept telling him over and over again that I was so sorry I couldn't carry his baby to term. He looked at me and told me it was okay and that he loved me, regardless of what happened. Shortly after, they pulled Bo from my womb and handed him to the neonatologist, whose staff had just finished preparing the baby bed warmer. My husband sat back down, looking very pale and sick. One of the nurses came over to make sure he was okay. During all this, the OR was loud. Once Bo was out, the room became totally silent, and I started asking my husband what was wrong. He told me they were working on Bo and putting me back together. The anesthesiologist came over and started to sedate me. I kept insisting that I had to see Bo before they took him to the NICU.

As soon as Bo was born, the neonatologist took over and intubated him with an endotrachial (ET) tube. He was also infused with Surfactant to help his lungs work properly. The ET tube breathed for him through a high-frequency oscillating ventilator (HFOV). In the delivery room he was also given epinephrine to increase his heart rate, which ranged between 60 and 80 beats per minute. His heart rate immediately began to rise, and he was taken to the Neonatal

Intensive Care Unit (NICU), but not before they allowed me to get a quick look at my new baby boy. Never had I seen such a tiny red baby, whose eyes were fused shut. My lasting impression was of his head, which was about the size of a tennis ball.

The doctors asked my husband if he wanted to stay with me or go with Bo. I told him to go with Bo and make sure he was going to be all right and that I would be fine. He came back shortly to report that Bo was doing as well as could be expected. The next thing I remember was being in the recovery room, with my mother wiping the hair from my eyes. I was confused about what had happened and wasn't sure where my husband was. My mother said he'd gone home to take the boys to school. On a side note, Cy, my stepson, didn't even remember our telling him that we were leaving for the hospital. When my husband told them they had a baby brother, neither one believed him and just assumed I was back in the hospital as I had been before. They became believers very shortly, however.

Bo was born weighing 1 pound 3 ounces (555 grams), was 8¼ inches long (21 centimeters), and was sixteen weeks early. About two hours after his birth I was able to see him. We were told that the first forty-eight hours were the most critical. My mother called our pastor immediately after Bo was born (5:14 A.M.), he rushed over to be with us, and we had him baptized immediately. We were so afraid that something would happen to take him away from us. One of the NICU nurses even told my mother that Bo would never be normal, something my mother did not share with me for a long time.

At birth Bo had very red and pink translucent skin. His eyes, fused shut (like a newborn puppy's eyes), did not open for about two weeks. He was covered in goop to keep his thin skin from drying out. He had two or three layers of skin on his little body; adults have around forty layers. The nurses had to be very careful because if his skin was simply rubbed, it could come off and scar him badly. He was kept under a little plastic-looking tent, again to keep in the moisture. They gave him a 20 percent chance to live. The week after the first forty-eight hours was the honeymoon period. After that first week, things could go any way. We did the preemie two-step—one step forward and two steps back—most of the time he was there.

During the first few days of Bo's life, I was still bedridden and wasn't able to go to the NICU to see him. I vaguely remember being furious with my mother and stepfather and resentful because they could see Bo as much as they wanted, while I had to lie in bed and wait for their reports. I felt they knew more about my son than I did. There were some very deep feelings those first few days. I wanted to see for myself that Bo was doing okay, but all I got were reports. Finally I was able to see with my own eyes how my precious, tiny baby was doing.

I was not able to hold Bo for almost two weeks, and when I did, it was only for about five minutes. When we went to visit, one of my favorite nurses told me not to have a heart attack but she was going to let me hold him. She ran around trying to find a Polaroid camera to capture the moment. After she handed him to me for the first time, my mom and I just stood there, crying and looking down at my beautiful son. Oh, what joy!

There were times when we couldn't touch or talk to him because he had apnea and brady spells. All we could do was look at him in the isolette. He had the normal problems that most premature infants have. At one week of age, he was diagnosed with a grade II intraventricular hermorrhage (brain bleed). The doctors kept a close watch on his IVH because it could cause problems (hydrocephalus) later. He had about seven head sonograms to make sure it was resolving. One day I went into the NICU and asked about his latest sonogram. The nurses were very guarded and said the doctors would have to compare it with his last one. I kept asking what that meant—was it good, bad, or what? They told me I shouldn't worry about it now because if what was suspected was the case, then I'd just have to deal with it. I was terrified. I racked my brain trying to remember what I'd read about these types of things and came up with only one that I thought was bad enough to cause such a reaction from the nurses. It was periventricular leukomalacia (PVL). I asked the nurses if that was what the concern was about, and they asked if I'd been talking to someone. I told them I'd been reading up on preemies and that PVL was something that could happen, and it would most likely cause cerebral palsy. Again, they told me not to think or read about it but to wait. This kind of advice from the nurses drove me crazy. I am a realist and want to know what problems I might be facing before the problems slap me in the face. So I went and read about PVL and panicked. The doctor said he didn't think it was PVL, but the IVH was actually a periventricular hemorrhage, which again threw me for a loop. Did this mean he had PVL? It was finally explained that the bleed had occurred outside of the ventricles instead of inside. An MRI was scheduled to rule it out before Bo could come home.

During this time the doctors were trying to get Bo's blood sugar levels straight. He had an IV drip of insulin to help this apparently common side effect of prematurity. He had about three suspected cases of sepsis, a blood infection, but thank goodness each time it was ruled out.

Bo started on expressed breast milk on August 19 by an oral gastrointestinal tube. They were able to increase the volume slowly, and he tolerated the milk well. About a month later his stomach became distended and firm. This was the only time that the hospital called us with frightening news. They said they were stopping the feedings for now and were going to watch him very closely. The doctors ordered an X ray, and it showed a lot of gas in his intestines. The good news was that it wasn't NEC, which could kill a premature baby. He resumed the feedings a couple of days later with a lower-calorie fortifier. On October 27, Bo was able to start bolus feedings, which is done by holding a syringe filled with milk that goes through his NG tube to his stomach. My husband I were taught to feed him that way and were finally enjoying "feeding" our son. During the bolus feed we gave him a pacifier so that he would associate sucking with getting a full belly. Finally, about a week or two later, we were able to introduce a bottle. He was diagnosed as a "poor nipple feeder." He worked his way up to about three bottles a day, and I was able to convince the doctors that I could gavage (bolus) him the rest at home. They agreed, and I was taught to insert the NG tube, listen for placement, and check for residuals. The funny thing is that a little over a week after he came home, he was taking all meals by bottle. I believe the nipples that the NICU used just weren't right for Bo, which is why he did so poorly.

I pumped breast milk for ten weeks and finally decided to quit. From the beginning I had trouble producing very much milk, and as Bo's needs increased, my output decreased. This was very frustrating because it seemed at the time that pumping was all I could do for my son. I experienced a lot of guilt over the decision to quit but soon realized I was a lot less stressed and could focus more on Bo.

Bo had ten blood transfusions for anemia due to prematurity. I became pretty knowledgeable about this and could tell when his eyelids became a deep blue or purple and his skin color was almost yellow. I would ask what his hematocrit level was, and they'd usually tell me it was very low and the blood had been ordered. I hated for him to have these transfusions, but I could sure tell the difference once they were done. One time an IV was put in Bo's scalp and blew the vein; he ended up with a big bruise mark on the side of his head. Another time they tried to place an IV in his scalp, and it also blew, so now I warn any nurse who wants to use his scalp veins. They still try it, though, and then I get to tell them, "I told you so." Finally, they decided to insert a central line IV, a permanent type of IV. Because Bo's skin was so thin and there was no way to tape the IV on really well, they inserted it in the artery in his neck. I was scared, but the surgery went without a hitch. Bo kept the central line in for about three weeks before it was removed because they weren't able to obtain any blood from it. He has a small scar on his right breast and on his neck, but with time they should be barely noticeable.

Because Bo gained weight very slowly, the doctors put him on MCT (medium chain triglycerides) oils to help him. He finally hit the 2-pound mark on September 26, about a month and a half later. I brought in a star with his weight and the date, and threw a "2-Pound Party." A little over a month later he hit 3 pounds, and we threw a "3-Pound Party" and gave him a star with the statistics of that day. His "4-Pound Party" came after he reached that weight on November 18. Friends from work wrote sayings and signed their names on his star for him to read when he gets older. My mother and I printed up cute signs each time and posted them over his bed. Fellow preemie parents and nurses said they enjoyed reading Bo's newest signs.

Bo was first intubated on August 14, was on the high-frequency ventilator (HFOV) for five days, and was then changed to the conventional mechanical ventilator, which he stayed on for almost a month and a half. On September 11 they extubated him and let him try the nasal CPAP (continuous positive airway pressure). One of my favorite nurses took three Polaroid pictures of him without all the tubing and tape all over his face. After a few hours he started desatting (blood oxygen levels went lower than desired). They intubated him again, and he stayed on it until September 26 when he was successfully extubated again and restarted on CPAP. Bo started Decadron (a steroid) due to recurrent bradycardia. He was weaned from this steroid about a month later. On November 8, he was changed to a nasal cannula. He kept pulling the cannula from his nose, and they decided to let him try breathing without assistance. He had to be restarted a couple of days later due to apnea with desaturation episodes and was finally able to breathe without assistance about four days later. Since he was on the vent for almost three months, he was diagnosed with chronic lung disease.

Bo was hooked up to many monitors for heart rate, breathing

rate, and blood oxygen levels. The alarms went off quite often and scared us to death at first. We finally became used to them and knew what to look for whenever one sounded. Sometimes it was very hard not to stare at the monitors and watch the numbers. My husband was the worst of all of us. One of the nurses suggested we watch Bo, not the monitors. "You can tell more from looking at the baby than you can from the monitors," she said. Bo had many alarms for apnea and bradycardia, and at one point was taking Doxapram and caffeine to regulate his breathing and heart rates. He came off those but went back on caffeine because he had trouble after being sedated for an MRI. He was on caffeine when he came home, but we were able to discontinue its use after a month.

Bo was diagnosed with very minor retinopathy of prematurity (ROP). After many eye exams, it was determined that it had resolved, and he didn't have any visual impairment.

One of my happiest days during his 104-day stay was when they allowed me to "kangaroo" him. Kangaroo care encourages skin-to-skin contact. I was able to lay Bo on my bare chest, with blankets draped over us. I was so thrilled when we did this. Bo handled it very well. His breathing became very regular, and his body temperature raised several degrees, a good sign that he was tolerating it. When he didn't tolerate it very well, it made me feel that he was rejecting me. He may have been overstimulated, tired, or any number of things. I couldn't help feeling bad when this happened, though. The kangarooing was increased to twice daily during the month of November. He tolerated it well and gained weight much better.

Before we were able to bring him home, we stayed at the hospital in a room that was directly across from the NICU and were given training on his apnea monitor. My husband and I were so nervous. We were afraid something would go wrong and they wouldn't let us take him home. We were afraid we would do something wrong that might damage him for life. He had been well taken care of in the

NICU, and now we were responsible! I felt fear like I've never known fear before!

The nurse brought Bo to the room and then left. My husband and I kept "fighting" over which one of us could hold him. If I lay Bo down, my husband would pick him up. I'd tell him Bo needed to lie in his crib. As soon as my husband would put him down, I'd find a reason to pick him up. I think it was the freedom from the nurse's eye that made us this way. We could finally do whatever we wanted to do with him, whenever we wanted. We hardly slept a wink that night, with each of us getting up a couple of times to check on him. His alarm never went off, which was really a blessing. If it had, we probably would have told the doctors to keep him a little longer! The next morning Bo was discharged. He weighed a whopping 4 pounds 8 ounces. He also got his picture taken by the newborn baby photographer. The nurse then put me in a wheelchair with Bo in my lap. She wheeled us to the NICU, and we said our good-byes with lots of hugs and kisses and good wishes. One of the nurses took a picture of our "going home day" to be put on the "graduates" picture board. She then wheeled us down to the car, with my husband taking pictures. We were so happy that day. All we'd ever wanted, dreamed of, and wished for had finally come true. We were going home.

Bo has now been home almost seven months. He has had one small cold, which was really just nasal stuffiness. He had five Respigam infusions from November to April to combat RSV. He has been gaining about 1 pound a month. At this time he weighs about 16 pounds and is about 24 inches long. He loves to eat baby food, and his favorites are sweet potatoes and corn. He's a very happy and healthy little guy. He has two bottom teeth and is currently working on his two canine (Dracula) teeth. He is probably going to have a really strange-looking smile soon!

Developmentally he's doing well. He rolls from stomach to back, and back to stomach. He still cannot sit up without support, but we are working on that. He babbles and says da-da, geh, nine-nine-nine (when he's really mad), and a couple of others. He does have tightness in his hamstrings and heel chords, so Early Intervention comes twice a month for therapy. E.I. tells us that he's ahead in his language skills and fine-motor skills but behind in gross-motor skills.

Bo is the light of my life. He has traveled such a long, hard road and is still the sweetest, most loving baby. He is a miracle, and it is such a joy and gift to watch him grow. Although our preemie road has not yet ended, I feel that Bo has given me the strength and courage to face any challenges that might come our way.

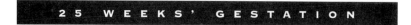

BABY BOY KING:
TOMMY'S STORY

by Clark T. King

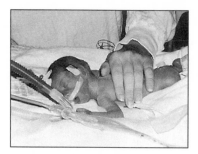

Thomas during early days in the NICU.

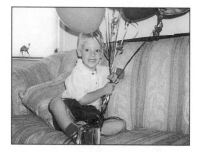

Thomas, four years old.

Thomas Clark King was born at 9:18 A.M. on July 26, 1994. I had taken his mother, Natalie Mary King, to the emergency room at approximately 8:30 A.M. on that same day. She had been having problems with vaginal bleeding and had been in and out of the hospital and doctor's office the week prior to Thomas's birth. Thomas's early birth was due to a placenta abruption, which occurs when the placenta separates from the uterus. (Thomas's placenta was separated approximately 75 percent.) When this occurs, a woman's body tends to deliver the baby in order to protect the mother and the baby, but it is a very dangerous situation because both can bleed to death. Having had various bleeding episodes the week before, Natalie chose not to wake me to let me know she was having a problem.

When I saw her in the morning, I was alarmed at her appearance and demanded that we go to the emergency room immediately.

After we arrived at the hospital and Natalie had been examined, we were told that she was 3 to 4 centimeters dilated and in labor. This was only five months into the pregnancy. When I was told she was in labor, I believed she was going to have a stillbirth because it was too early for the baby to survive. What followed was the most frightening and amazing experience we had ever encountered. We were told that, yes, babies born at twenty-five weeks do survive and that the hospital staff was going to do everything in their power to save our baby. Natalie was prepared for surgery (in case a cesarean was necessary), and I put on scrubs. She was taken to the delivery room with me in tow.

In the delivery room it was determined that the baby's presentation was wrong and that he would have to be taken by emergency cesarean. I was escorted out of the delivery room and left in the hallway to wait. After what seemed like an eternity, I was told that the baby would be coming soon and that I should wait close to the main hallway. The team that took him out of the delivery room brought him out in a transport cart headed for the Neonatal Intensive Care Unit (NICU). The neonatologist who had been present for the delivery allowed them to stop briefly for my first view of my tiny son. He had been intubated in the delivery room and was the smallest and most sickly baby I had ever seen.

After Baby Boy King had been taken to the NICU and stabilized, the neonatologist took me for my first visit to what would become very familiar territory for me and my family over the next four months, the Neonatal Intensive Care Unit. I was instructed on the hand-washing procedure that would become second nature to me. I was introduced to the yellow gown required over my clothing prior to entry and was then taken into room two of the NICU. No one could be prepared for what had happened to us that day. I certainly was not prepared to become a father just over halfway through the pregnancy.

The baby I was taken to was like none I had ever known could survive. However, he was my son, and I was doing my best to take on the role of his father. I asked if I could touch him and was told to go ahead. I touched my index finger to his little hand, and he grabbed the tip of my finger. His hand was too small to grab anything more.

The neonatologist brought me two pictures they had taken of him and asked if she should bring them to my wife. The pictures made him look even worse than he did, and I asked that another picture be taken for me to bring to Natalie. My mission at that point was to find my wife and give our baby a name. If I could give him nothing else, I could give him a name. Natalie asked that we name him Thomas because she knew that was my preference. We named him Thomas Clark King after me, his father, Clark Thompson King. He is the fourth generation of King men with Clark in his name.

Thomas in the NICU

We were told that six or seven out of ten babies born at twenty-five weeks survive. Of those who don't survive, most are lost within the first forty-eight hours. Thomas did well not just for that forty-eight hours but for the next week. Preemies who survive tend to go through what is called a "honeymoon period" where things tend to go very well before any real decline is seen. It is during this period of about a week that the baby adjusts to life outside the womb. We were warned that things were likely to get much worse before they got better.

Thomas had an excellent honeymoon period. Although he was on a respirator and would be for the next several weeks, his settings were fairly low compared to what they could have been. On Friday of the week of his birth (he was born on Tuesday), his mother and I were even allowed to hold him a little bit, respirator tubes and all. About a week after his birth we encountered some problems. Thomas had been getting blood transfusions to replace the blood that was constantly being drawn for lab tests. After taking his blood, it was noticed that the wound would continue to bleed beyond what was liked by the health care professionals. Although it wasn't a major concern, we were asked for family history in this area.

During the second week, Thomas had a brain bleed (intraventricular hemorrhage). Although quite common in preemies, especially extremely premature babies like Thomas, it was rather disconcerting. Many of the major handicaps of preemies seem to be traced back to these brain bleeds. Fortunately, Thomas's bleed was said to be fairly minor (a grade I intraventricular hemorrhage). Normal room air is approximately 21 percent oxygen. Thomas's respirator oxygen requirements had tended to range from the 20s to the 40s during his first couple of weeks. During the third week his requirements increased to the 60 percent and up to the 90 percent range. Thomas was put on antibiotics as a precaution and tested for infection. Although the twenty-four- and forty-eight-hour cultures were negative, the seventy-two-hour culture came back positive. The antibiotics were continued, and we had a nervous few days.

The doctors decided to use steroids (Decadron) to see if that would ease his oxygen requirements. We were warned that he would be fussier on the steroids and would continue to dislike being touched. Since he had been sick, he was unable to handle our touch very often. From the very beginning we had been encouraged to visit, talk to him, and carefully touch him. (My wife visited every single day of his four-month hospitalization, and I missed only five days.) Preemies have an immature nervous system that can only handle one thing at a time, so we were encouraged to approach him slowly with only one sensation at a time. The steroid had the appropriate effect: His oxygen requirements went back down, the pressure and rate settings were set less aggressively, and he seemed much better during his fourth week.

Around this time Natalie and I learned what a "brady" spell is. A brady, or bradycardia, is when the heart rate falls below 100. It usually is related to a "desat," or desaturation, where the oxygenation of the blood falls and stays below 85. Usually a brady follows an apnea spell, which is when he forgets to breathe for fifteen seconds or more. As long as Thomas was on a respirator, those spells weren't a great concern. The attentive nursing staff would turn his oxygen up (to 100 percent if necessary) or occasionally "bag" him with a hand pump that forced air into his lungs. His mother and I became accustomed to these spells; however, other family members found them very disconcerting. When you saw these episodes every day and were assured by the nursing staff that they were par for the course, you stopped being alarmed—as long as he was properly attended to by the staff. As our comfort level in the NICU increased, we even assisted the staff by stimulating him: A pat on the back or behind would usually remind him to breathe, or we would turn up the oxygen according to the staff's instructions.

Life in the NICU

We became very familiar, even comfortable, with the NICU during Thomas's four-month stay. We assisted with the feedings and with anything else the staff allowed us to do. We learned what to watch for and what to ignore on the monitors that he was connected to twenty-four hours a day. Basically we learned how to be NICU parents following the example set by other parents we saw in the NICU.

Thomas was fed breast milk through a small tube. The tube was passed down his throat directly into Thomas's stomach. Babies at this stage have no gag reflex, so it is not thought to be uncomfortable for them. At this stage he was too immature to be able to suck, swallow, or breathe the way a more mature baby would to accomplish eating. When Thomas was first born, we were told of the advantages of feeding preemies breast milk and encouraged to provide it for him. Natalie rented a special breast pump and began pumping her breasts every three or four hours. She was instructed to save all of it even if she only produced a little. The milk was marked with Thomas's name and the date, then frozen and put into storage. My wife's persistence made it possible for Thomas to receive breast milk exclusively for the first seven and a half months of his life.

Having a baby in the hospital completely disrupts your life. Almost every night of the week we ate out, ordered takeout, or ate one of the care packages we received from well wishers. We had little time for normal things like cooking dinner. We used to make light of the situation and joke that we had the best day care money could buy and could still go out anytime we wanted. What we really wanted, of course, was a healthy baby and a return to a somewhat normal life.

For the first ten weeks of Thomas's life his mother was on maternity leave and able to devote herself to Thomas 100 percent. Knowing she was at the hospital very day made it easier for me to go to work. I knew she would call with updates and progress reports if anything exciting happened. Every day after work I went directly to the hospital and stayed for about an hour or so. We found the first five weeks of Thomas's hospitalization the hardest. He gained weight very slowly after dropping to as low as 1 pound 6 ounces two days after his birth. People would constantly ask if he weighed 2 pounds yet. Our answer was always no. We were assured by the nursing staff that he was doing great and that progress would come before we knew it. We knew they had seen this all before and tried to trust what they were telling us. They were right, of course, but it was hard to believe it at the time.

Tommy Gets off the Respirator

Thomas turned five weeks old on August 30, 1994. At 11:55 A.M. that day he was extubated from the respirator for the very first time and placed under an oxygen hood to receive supplemental oxygen. For the first time he was breathing with no mechanical assistance, an exciting step in his development. We were finally able to see his cute little face without the respirator tube obstructing our view. It appeared that progress was being made. Thomas remained off the respirator for seventeen hours before he was reintubated. It was thought that he was struggling and still in need of the support provided by the respirator. However, we were told beforehand that this would probably be the case. He was to be reintubated for a while and then tested off the respirator again when he seemed strong enough.

On September 3, 1994, Thomas reached another milestone: He finally achieved 2 pounds. His primary nurse gave him the coveted "2-pound award for his unbelievable weight achievement," and we could finally tell people that he weighed over 2 pounds.

The nurses in the NICU provide most of the care that the babies receive while in the NICU. At many hospitals they assign a primary nurse who is the primary caretaker for several infants while on duty. The primary nurse usually becomes a friend and advocate for the parents. We found this system quite helpful and are still in contact with Thomas's primary nurse. One of the neat things the nurses of the NICU do for the family is help prepare a journal with Polaroid photographs and enhance the photographs with special comments. Parents and relatives are encouraged to write in the book as well. Comments from Tommy's book include:

> Hi Mommy & Daddy—I know I came earlier than expected, but I'm doing good & I'm a little fighter!

> I'm so cute & my nurses think I'm real strong because I turned my head 3 times today.

> Hi! It must be 2 A.M. again cuz I'm wide awake!

> Me & Mommy look so happy together! I love when she holds me!

> That's me, Daddy & Grandpa! Three generations of us King men! (I'm the cute one.)

> I can't wait to eat all that good Polish food I heard Grandpa [Gladysz] talking about.

Tommy Extubates Himself

Monday, September 5, 1994, began the week in which Tommy's doctors pretty much decided to let him coast for a little while before trying anything new. Tommy evidently had a different view of what was to come next. Much to the dismay of the staff, on Thursday, September 8, he extubated himself from the respirator. Rather than reintubate a little fighter who obviously knew what was best, he was put on a less aggressive nasal CPAP (pronounced C-pap, and it means continuous positive airway pressure). Unlike a respirator, the CPAP doesn't actually mechanically breathe for the baby but provides continuous air pressure that makes it easier for the baby to inflate his or her lungs when inhaling. It is less aggressive and less invasive than the respirator.

On that Sunday, September 11, after a successful few days on the CPAP, Thomas was once again put under an oxygen hood. He handled the oxygen hood much better this time and stayed off more aggressive support for a long while. Shortly after he was put under the oxygen hood, his mother and I went to visit. His primary nurse was on duty and asked if we wanted to hold him. We had been allowed to hold him from time to time but always for very short periods and with the staff attending to the invasive respiratory equipment he required. On that day we were both able to hold him with only a hose blowing supplemental oxygen across his face. It was wonderful. We were told that babies who are held and handled by their parents do better than those who were left alone. NICU babies are necessarily poked and prodded by the staff so much that human touch is not always pleasant for them. As NICU parents it was our job to give him love through gentle and cautious touching. It was also our job to give him something pleasant in his life when not much was pleasant for him. We were sure to hold him and touch him as much as we could; it was one of the very few things we could do that made us feel like his parents.

After we left that evening, Thomas was moved from his warming table to an isolette incubator. Extremely premature babies requiring constant care are kept openly exposed on a warming table that provides easy access to the staff in case a situation arises. More mature preemies who require less constant attention benefit from the isolation and relative quiet available inside the isolette. It also shields them from airborne germs. NICUs are noisy places. Each baby is connected to a pulse oximeter to measure the oxygen in their blood and a respiratory and heart rate monitor. These monitors go off frequently and are constantly observed by the staff. A beeping monitor was usually nothing to panic about. It generally signified a false alarm, a warning that something needed to be adjusted, or a warning that the baby needed some brief attention.

Four Months Is a Long Time

One of the most frightening things about the day Thomas was born was knowing that his survival would require several weeks of hospitalization. His progress over the first six weeks of that hospitalization assured us that he would most likely survive and that he had a very good chance of escaping major disabilities. It was after Tommy was permanently taken off the respirator and moved to the isolette that this hospital stay started to feel like a drawn-out waiting game and began to weigh on us. After a week of having just about the healthiest baby in room two, we were moved to room five for babies requiring somewhat less intensive care. We went from having one of the healthiest babies in the room to one in which he was about the least healthy. Moving from room two to room five introduced us to a slightly different set of nurses. Some were—appropriately—far more critical of our handling of Thomas while we were visiting. Since were permitted to handle and hold him on a regular basis, there was more to criticize. This really began our education as parents of a preemie. Where before we were more like spectators than participants, now we were trying to take a more active part in his care.

The NICU experience is described as "two steps forward and one step back." Up to this point we felt that we'd taken many more steps forward than steps back. Unfortunately, week eight included a step back. Thomas's oxygen requirements went up, and he became more sensitive to being handled. He had been put back on the CPAP, placed on antibiotics, and was being tested for infection. Once again, negative twenty-four- and forty-eight-hour cultures were followed by a positive culture at seventy-two hours. It was decided that Thomas required more intensive care than what was available in room five, so he was moved to room three. It was a hard step back for his parents. Thomas improved after about a week, just in time to receive his 3-pound award.

After her ten weeks of leave, Natalie finally had to return to work. It was difficult for her because she knew it would be harder to spend time with him every day. The night before Natalie returned to work, we went for an extended Sunday night visit in which we were permitted to bathe him together for the first time. The day Natalie returned to work, she received a flower arrangement from Thomas with a note: "Daddy says you have to go to work to buy me lots of toys. Go to it, Mom!" To this day I don't know how Thomas borrowed the credit card!

Thomas Learns to Breast-Feed

Around the gestational age of thirty-four weeks, babies are capable of the suck, swallow, and breathe pattern, enabling them to take food more normally. The goal at this point is to get them accustomed to the bottle and get them off tube feedings. It was around this age and shortly after Natalie returned to work that she gave Thomas his first bottle. He went from being exclusively tube fed to receiving milk via the bottle every so many feedings. After having mastered bottle feeding, it eventually became time for Thomas to move on to other things. Here is a description of that experience by Thomas's mother:

> Soon after delivery the possibility of breast-feeding was discussed. Although Thomas would be unable to feed directly from the breast at first, the milk could be expressed and frozen for use as necessary. It was strongly encouraged for mothers to provide breast milk to the premature babies. This being the case and knowing I couldn't do much else for Thomas, I decided to give it a try. After being attached to a mechanical breast pump for 2½ months, I looked forward to the day when I could feed Thomas naturally. Before Thomas and I made our first attempt at breast-feeding, we experimented with a little skin-to-skin contact. Thomas's father and I had read about the concept of "kangaroo care," which is the practice of the mother kangaroo holding her baby (called a joey) next to her bare chest in her pouch. Kangaroo care has been found to help nurture premature babies through the NICU experience. It was our experimentation with skin-to-skin kangaroo care that led to our first try at breast-feeding. The first time Thomas latched on to my breast was by accident during a skin-to-skin experience. Thomas latched on and ended up with a mouthful of milk he didn't expect and wasn't prepared for! Although we had a lot of ground to cover, it was wonderful to finally be approaching this milestone. The first time I actually tried to feed Thomas, it was quite a struggle. He wanted the instant gratification of the bottle and didn't have the patience to wait for me to let down. That time and many a time thereafter I left the NICU feeling disappointed that he didn't want me and that I wasn't a good mother. These trials and tribulations frustrated both of us. He had mastered the bottle and was apparently confused and frustrated when we

asked him to try something different. Fortunately, the NICU nurses were fantastic with their persistence and coaching efforts and helped us be successful much of the time. Once I resigned myself to the fact that it would get better when I fed Thomas all the time, I felt I wasn't failing him in some way. It was a time of learning for both of us.

Most mothers and babies don't have to learn breast-feeding behind a screen in a busy NICU. Natalie deserves credit for her persistence that continued even when Thomas refused the breast in favor of the bottle. Eventually he overcame his "nipple confusion" and became an effective breast-feeder. However, that didn't and couldn't happen until he was released from the NICU.

The Waiting Game Continues

When Thomas was born, we were told that preemies tend to go home around their due date. As Thomas's November 6 due date approached, it became apparent that he would not be going home that soon. Things were going well, and there were fewer and fewer concerns. He was gaining weight, gradually improving every day, and looking and acting more and more like a normal baby. The two key concerns were his eyes and his oxygen requirements. As is common with extremely premature babies, Thomas had ROP (retinopathy of prematurity), which can cause varying degrees of visual impairment. Fortunately, many advances are being made in the treatment of ROP. Thomas, at one point, was scheduled for laser surgery to avoid a detached retina due to his ROP. Just days before, sufficient improvement was discovered, and the surgery was canceled. Thomas was seen by a specialist for a short period even after he was released from the hospital. Fortunately, no lasting vision problem has been detected as of a year later.

The other concern was his oxygen requirements. Early on, Thomas's bronchopulmonary dysplasia (BPD) was treated through intubation on a respirator. After the respirator and CPAP were no longer required, months of oxygen therapy were necessary to allow the lungs to mature and heal from the previous treatments. The goal was to lessen his oxygen requirements to enable him to go home. Mostly it was a long waiting game.

Our families and friends were very supportive through this period as well as throughout the entire hospitalization and its aftermath. Thomas's grandparents visited the NICU as often as they could, as did his aunts and uncles. Their support was and is important to us. Although we were permitted to bring in others, we felt we should limit visitors to immediate family in order to expose Thomas to fewer outside germs and also avoid having to explain what was happening within the NICU environment. Although you become accustomed to it, first visits to a NICU are shocking, and most people have never seen anything like it. We also appreciated the camaraderie that formed between us and many of the other NICU parents. We were asked not to inquire too much about the other babies, families, and so forth, but you can't spend four months seeing many of the same faces on a regular basis without forming some type of relationship. I remember congratulating parents upon hearing of their release dates and improvements. I also remember some very bad days in the NICU I don't want to talk about.

Tommy Goes Home!

It was the Tuesday before Thanksgiving when we finally got the word: Thomas was going home! It would be on Monday or Tuesday of the following week. We found ourselves unprepared for the very event we had been longing for. We suddenly realized we would have to juggle work schedules and prepare for his homecoming.

The game plan was as follows: Wednesday, receive infant CPR and first aid training and learn how to use the home oxygen equipment and monitors (apnea monitor and pulse oximeter); Thursday, learn what medications he was to take, when he was to take them, and how to administer them (and afterward eat turkey); Friday, make sure we could handle him on our own by staying overnight with Thomas completely in our care in a private room at the hospital with the hospital staff available if needed; Saturday, review any questions regarding the overnight stay with the staff; Sunday, prepare our house to receive Thomas (the required equipment had been delivered Friday); Monday, last-minute preparations; Tuesday, assuming a final okay from his doctors, especially from the eye specialist who would be seeing him regularly for a little while, Tommy would go home.

We made the appropriate arrangements with our employers and became incredibly excited about Tommy's going home. Wednesday's training was a breeze because we had had four months of NICU parenting under our belt and were not intimidated by the equipment we would be using. We spent a very happy Thanksgiving day in the NICU going over Tommy's medication, thanking his primary nurse for everything she had done, and receiving congratulations from the other NICU parents (most of whom would be following us very shortly). We left late in the afternoon, in time for Thanksgiving dinner. The overnight stay at the hospital went fine. We even managed to get some sleep between false monitor alarms. With just the three of us in the hospital room together, we finally got to spend time alone as a family. We were ready to take him home.

Tuesday finally came. We went out to breakfast (it would be a while before we could do that again) and proceeded to the hospital to bring him home. Tommy received the okay from his doctors and was homeward bound.

Thomas at Home on Oxygen

We had three oxygen tanks to use at home with Thomas: an over-the-shoulder portable tank for traveling home from the hospital and to doctor appointments, a slightly larger tank on wheels for use around the house, and a huge green tank that became the largest single decoration in his nursery. We also had a pulse oximeter and an apnea monitor, although the apnea monitor was really just a safeguard in case the pulse oximeter failed and the nasal cannula came out of place. With the oxygen came hoses (fifty feet and ten feet) to connect the tanks and the cannula; with the fifty-foot hose we could take Thomas through most of the downstairs and still have him connected to the tank in his bedroom.

Thomas's mother, grandmother, and I had received training in all the equipment. Other family members were to be trained as necessary to be caregivers. No one outside the family was permitted in the house until spring. We elected to keep even family members away for the first twenty-four hours, which allowed us to familiarize ourselves with the equipment and to develop routines with Tommy's feedings and the medications he was to continue at home (diuretics and vitamins). After four months as NICU parents, we found it easier than we expected to fall into a routine at home. Since all he really did at this point was sleep and eat (he was equivalent to a one-month-old in development), there didn't seem much to it. The easiest thing to remember was the continuous hand washing—a routine we developed in the NICU because the doctors felt it was so important. The hardest part was the monitors. Most of the alarms they emit are false alarms caused by misplaced leads or simple movement by the baby; however, it is important to look at the baby to make sure everything is okay. In the NICU, nurses are awake and ready to check the alarms as needed. At 3 A.M., Natalie and I were generally not awake. Between false monitor alarms and a baby who breast-fed every two hours, our sleeping patterns were completely disrupted. We were informed more times than was appreciated that interrupted sleeping patterns are normal for new parents, but most new parents don't have to wake up to make sure a cannula is in place, the oxygen is functioning, and that there isn't an extraordinary emergency situation developing. And while every parent worries that everything is okay, most don't have a high-risk, special-needs infant to be concerned about.

Around Valentine's Day we had an appointment with the neona-tologist, who agreed Thomas was ready to be removed from the oxy-gen; however, the oxygen and monitors were to remain in the house until things seemed all clear. On Palm Sunday we took Thomas to church for his first outing. We also relaxed visiting restrictions, al-though we did ask everyone to wash their hands before handling him. On May 7, 1995, Thomas was welcomed by the church (we had had him baptized the day he was born), and a christening party introduced him to the entire family. It was time to begin a more nor-mal life.

Two Years Later

As I write this, Tommy is just shy of two years and eleven months old, and a little over two years and six months corrected (although we only rarely consider his corrected age at this point). In about a month he will become a big brother. Although small for his age, Tommy seems very much the normal two-and-a-half-year-old. Last month he started sleeping in his "big boy bed." He is constantly sur-prising me with his speech, which is becoming more and more con-versational. "I can do it" is replacing "no" as a frequent utterance even when his parents would prefer he didn't do it!

When Tommy was born, I had very little hope that we would ever get to this point. The NICU is such an unreal place and the infor-mation on micropreemies is so grim that I couldn't see beyond the horror of Tommy's early birth—fifteen weeks early and 1 pound 10 ounces. I've learned a lot since then. Micropreemies can have posi-tive outcomes. Some of these babies will have few or no problems; a greater percentage than anyone likes will have minor disabilities; and some will have serious problems. However, even a child with disabilities can have a full life and can be considered a positive outcome! I've also learned that babies born just one or two months early or even at term can have serious problems, although their problems are dismissed while the negative outcomes of micropreemies are amplified. The horror of an early birth is not just a matter of outcomes. It is a matter of a tiny baby who has lost the benefit of the ideal growing environment and faces challenges that most babies don't. It's a matter of losing a portion of the pregnancy as well as the perfect television birth where the doctor asks for one last push, announces it's a boy or girl, and the camera fades out on mother, father, and baby bonding for the first time. The fantasy moment is lost regardless of whether the baby is fifteen weeks early, ten weeks early, or even four weeks early.

It's difficult to understand the feeling of loss if you haven't been there. It's typical for well-meaning acquaintances to tell the mother of the preemie how she is lucky she "didn't get so big and have to go through those last few months of pregnancy" or "didn't have to deliver vaginally which hurts like hell." Well, my wife is loving the third trimester of her current pregnancy. Although we are parents, she has never been this pregnant before and cherishes every day of it. She also cries when she sees the television moment I described earlier because she knows that's not what we had with Tommy.

A 1977 MIRACLE:
SARA'S WILL TO LIVE

by Sally Stromseth

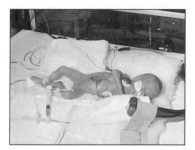

Sara, three days old.

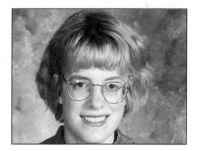

Sara, twenty-one years old.

We were so thankful to be pregnant again. Our first child had miscarried a year before at five and a half months and had left us devastated. We understood that miscarriages like mine were not common and that the chances of its happening again were slim. Even so, the grief over our loss was enough to keep us from even thinking about trying again for a while. What joy to know that a new baby was on the way. We were apprehensive but hopeful. I'd always had a big organic garden, so I felt sure that my diet was as good as possible. That, along with all the fresh air and exercise our Iowa farm life provided, was a prescription for a healthy pregnancy. My monthly trip to the doctor showed steady growth and weight gain. Then the momentous day finally came when I felt movement for the first time. That first tiny little flutter of feeling gave us hope beyond belief. As we neared the fifth month we were apprehensive. If we could just get beyond the gestation of my miscarriage, all would be well.

The fifth month arrived, and my appointment with the doctor showed that I'd started to dilate. We became very nervous. The pathologist's report a year before had determined my miscarriage was a result of an abnormality in the fetal spinal column. Any other possibilities, to my knowledge, were dismissed. We talked about my mom having taken the estrogen DES in 1949 when she was pregnant with me. Apparently I almost miscarried as a very young fetus, and it was common to give women DES to stop bleeding and possible miscarriage. Twenty years later those female babies exposed to DES reached childbearing years and suffered from an incompetent cervix. When gestation reached about the fifth to sixth month, the weak cervix would dilate with the increased weight of the baby, and the pregnancy would end in a late miscarriage or extremely premature delivery. A baby arriving in the fifth month at that time wasn't given even a remote chance of surviving. The six-month gestation survival rate was not encouraging, either.

Our doctor explained that minor surgery would be needed to stitch the cervix shut until the baby reached term. He sent us to a major medical facility sixty miles away to have a cerclage, a purse-string stitch, performed that literally prevented the baby from falling out of my uterus. Three days later, with no hint of early labor as a result of the surgery, I went home. My husband, Don, and I were encouraged to resume our lives. My activity level was, at best, limited and cautious. The doctors said I should be careful but not overreact. Well, I wouldn't even change a lightbulb because I thought reaching up too high might not be wise. As time went on and nothing horrible happened, I began to calm down.

My short daily walks provided not only fresh air and mild exercise but a daily dose of tranquility. As I crossed the bridge over the creek that runs through our pasture, and listened to the water rippling and the birds chirping, I was in awe of the beauty of it all. How lucky, I thought, to raise a family in such a wonderful place. What fun our children would have wading in the creek, picking wildflower bouquets, and listening to the frogs sing at night. As I walked on, I suddenly became aware of a wetness. It sent a horrified panic through me. Trying to keep my movements under control, I carefully made my way home, with tears easily getting the better of me. Fortunately, Don was working close by and helped me into the house. A phone call to the doctor had us packing for a trip to the hospital again. I lay down on the backseat of the car all the way to the hospital, slowly leaking what I presumed was amniotic fluid. My prayers from the start of my pregnancy had been to deliver a full-term, healthy, normal child. That trip was one long prayer for help.

When we arrived at the hospital, the emergency room staff was waiting for me. After running a couple of tests, it was determined that I was indeed leaking amniotic fluid. I was admitted to the hospital for bed rest in the hope that all would stop and right itself. They would keep me for a week and then send me home to continue constant bed rest until I delivered. I was at twenty-five weeks of gestation. All week long I leaked amniotic fluid, but the baby and I held our own. The heartbeat was strong, and no signs of early labor or distress were evident. The doctors said the baby would keep growing even in the absence of amniotic fluid. They were still hopeful, which made us hopeful. During that week I had three different roommates. Two of them were mothers of premature babies, born at longer gestations than my pregnancy was at the time. We each formed a bond in our short stay together. My third roommate was a very young unwed mother who was considering giving her baby up for adoption.

The end of the week arrived, and plans were in the works for my return home for continued bed rest. My parents were to drive a station wagon from their home to the hospital to take me home in a reclined position. Mom was prepared to stay as long as she was needed.

Between my parents and Don's, who lived in the next house down the road, I figured this could work.

When the nurse came in at 5:30 the next morning to do the usual checking, I complained of abdominal discomfort. A while later I was wheeled into a labor room to wait and see what would happen. My parents and in-laws were called. My mother-in-law later told me that the nurse who called her said they thought the mother could be saved but not the baby, so Don should come right away. After recovering from the initial shock of such a phone call, Don was fetched from the hay field and sent on his way.

The wait in the labor room was probably the loneliest time I'd ever spent in my life. The nurses were very kind and did what they could, but it seemed that our baby was going to be born at twenty-six weeks' gestation. I'd been told that a team of six neonatologists were on hand to take care of the baby if it was born alive. All this information seemed to get muddled in my head as I struggled to make some sense of our situation. How could things go wrong now after we'd tried so hard to do everything right?

I'd been praying constantly during the previous week, asking for strength and endurance for our unborn child. By the time I'd started labor I was already so tired from having been in bed all week that my reserves, both physical and mental, were taxed. My anxiety and desperation were at a peak as I continued to labor. At one point during the morning, the gynecologist who had initially examined me and ordered the surgery poked his head through the door. "Don't expect much," he said. "Your baby probably won't survive," and he shut the door. I was filled with such anger at his abrupt statement and lack of compassion that chasing him down the hallway hurling my IV at him was clearly a possibility, though remote.

Except for periodic checks, I was alone in the room. Don and my parents were on their way. My prayers turned from asking for help to asking for calm and grace to accept whatever happened. We had done all we could to save our child, so it was in God's hands now, as it had been from the start. I desperately needed to give Him this burden, so I did. Immediately, a sense of overwhelming calm came over me. The room felt warm, and I knew the presence of Jesus by my side. He literally held my hand until Don came.

Sara was born at 1:43 the following morning. At delivery she was whisked away to an adjoining room so fast by a neonatologist that the doctor delivering her was uncertain of her gender. All he could say was that the baby had taken a few breaths. Moments seemed like an eternity as the doctor worked on me and we waited for word from the other room. Suddenly I heard a faint cry through the closed door. Halfway sitting up, I asked if anyone else had heard it. Yes, what a joyful sound we'd all heard! A nurse came to me soon after to tell me that our little girl was kicking and screaming, and they were doing all they could to keep her that way. The nurse then went out to the waiting room to deliver the news to a very anxious daddy who was wearing out the carpet. How thankful we were to be surrounded by many caring and professional people, and yet how cheated we felt to go through all the motions of childbirth with no baby to hold.

At 7:30 A.M. a nurse came to my room to discuss Sara's condition. Her weight was recorded at 880 grams, which didn't mean anything to me. However, 1 pound 15 ounces meant a great deal! Her length was 14 inches. The biggest concern would be the state of her lungs, which weren't developed enough this early to do the job of breathing. The nurse explained that the events during the previous week of bed rest and leaking were to her advantage. Evidently a chemical reaction takes place, a warning to the baby that things are amiss so she should hurry up and develop her lungs. It was all so amazing. She was breathing on her own using no respirator but getting 35 percent oxygen through a tube to her nose. By evening the oxygen had increased to 43 percent, and she remained stable. We were given Sara's phone number to call at any time, day or night. How bizarre, we thought, to be given our infant daughter's phone number when we hadn't even seen her or held her for more than three minutes!

My parents had arrived during the early morning hours and came to see us by midmorning. They said they had checked in at a motel at 2 A.M. The lady who checked them in said she would pray for our little Sara. Don and my folks went to visit Sara for the first time, obviously without me. When they came back, the report was that she was tiny and beautiful, perfectly formed in every way and hooked up to machines with wires everywhere. We were all so tired that resting was necessary, especially for Don who had been up all night, too.

The next morning the supervising nurse reported that Sara's bilirubin level was up. Bilirubin, she explained, was a reddish-yellow pigment in the blood. The liver removes bilirubin from the bloodstream when everything is working right. In a tiny premature baby, bilirubin is quite common until the baby's liver develops enough to do its job properly. As a result of this, Sara would appear to be a little yellow in color. A test at 11:00 that morning would determine if she needed a blood transfusion. The nurse also explained that the first forty-eight hours were very critical. Initially, premature babies have energy to cope with their new environment, but later they begin to tire. Maintaining their body temperature, breathing, digesting, and putting up with IV leads and constant light and noise require a tremendous amount of energy that a normal full-term baby would have no trouble handling. If Sara could get through the first forty-eight hours, then the next milestone would be seventy-two hours, then a week, and so forth. One hour at a time and sometimes one minute at a time was a major step toward survival. All this information seemed so clinical that sometimes we'd forget we were actually talking about a living human being, our very own little daughter whom we loved. I decided to keep a journal so that I could digest all this again during the day and try to understand better how things were going.

By early afternoon a blood transfusion was started. It took ninety minutes to complete, during which Sara was closely monitored. A total of 10 centimeters of blood, 10 percent of her total blood volume, was taken out and 10 centimeters of new blood put in. Her bilirubin level was 8.2, which required the transfusion, whereas full-term babies could get up to a 20-point level before an exchange was necessary. By 5 P.M. the level had decreased to 5, and the oxygen in a tent over her little head was at 46 percent. Sara was on a flat open bed with lights above her to keep her bilirubin level down. The lights were so bright that the nurses covered her eyes to protect them. The lights can also dehydrate a baby, so Sara's arms and legs were covered with plastic wrap to help her retain her body fluids. She was getting 10 centimeters of glucose water every hour for three hours, and then she rested the fourth hour. A tube through her nose to her tummy was used to extract any remaining fluid to see how much she'd digested. It was explained that the open bed allowed her caregivers to get to all parts of the baby and the many tubes as quickly and efficiently as possible. She would eventually graduate to an incubator.

Don had to go home. The farmwork was very demanding, and he knew we were in good hands. Thankfully, we were only sixty miles apart, so visits could be frequent. By evening I started running a temperature and was put on antibiotics. What a revolting turn of events! I couldn't be released from the hospital until I'd been without a fever for twenty-four hours. Sara was twenty-four hours old in a hospital all hooked up to monitors and fighting to live; I was in a hospital down the road with a stupid fever, and Don was on the farm sixty miles away. What kind of family life was this? I needed to be near my baby, to hold and touch her. I couldn't even remember what she looked like, what color her hair was, or anything, just that she was tiny.

By the morning of the second day Sara was tiring. She would forget to breathe and have to be stimulated by tapping her foot to wake her up. To give her the rest she needed, the doctors put her on a respirator. They seemed to be satisfied with her activity level but decided to discontinue feeding her after two hours because it seemed to make her breathe heavier. We were reassured that it was normal for a baby to tire like this in a couple of days. Sara's weight had dropped to 1 pound 12½ ounces.

A new mom usually has her hands full with cuddling, feedings, and diapers. All I had was a visiting nurse, a phone number to Sara's room, and a journal. The one thing I could do was send colostrum to my child. On the day of her birth I asked for a breast pump so I could help some, but the request was lost or ignored. By the second day, after much reminding, I was given a pump. Not much could be expressed, but she didn't need much. So far I was keeping up with her needs. Later they would try to feed her a drop at a time through her feeding tube.

The first twenty-four hours had passed and then the next forty-eight hours. They gave her blood as needed to replace what they took for tests. The bilirubin level was at 6.9, and her breathing was more even. She started tolerating my colostrum, which made me feel more like a mom. I was actually feeding my baby long-distance. My temperature was still bothersome. Antibiotics plus enough water to make me slosh when I walked was all I could do. Daily phone calls from Don helped us keep our lives as even as possible. He had been haying and would come for a visit to see us both in the morning after chores. By 2 P.M. of the third day, Don was visiting Sara. She was able to digest 12 centimeters of colostrum (2 centimeters six times a day), and the bililights were off for a while. She opened her eyes and waved at her daddy. I could well imagine what that must have been like for him. "She's still small," he told me later.

The next day, when I had been twenty-four hours without a fever, I was discharged from the hospital. Mom and Dad had come back because Don was taking wedding pictures, our off-the-farm sideline, and couldn't ask the couple to change their wedding date this late. We went over to the hospital for my first visit since Sara's birth. I was scared and anxious at the same time. The NICU was behind closed double doors at the end of a long pediatric floor. We were instructed to scrub up to the elbows, take off our watches, and put on a gown before entering the room. Contamination from careless washing could prove tragic for ones so young and vulnerable.

Mom and Dad had warned me that Sara was still very small, trying to prepare me. All I could think of was that I could be with my child, look at her sweet face and talk to her. The nurse found a chair for me to use and led me to her open bed. The sight of her filled my eyes with tears. I just couldn't take it all in fast enough. She was so beautiful and fragile-looking. A fluff of light sandy hair, ears that looked like the most fragile of seashells, and long, delicately expressive fingers. I touched her hand, and immediately her fingers closed over mine with a tiny baby grip. We were bonded.

Through the course of the afternoon the nurse let me change her diaper three times. This involved folding a preemie disposable diaper in half and laying it under her little bottom. She didn't even wear clothes yet because it was vital to see all her body parts and where the leads connected. I cleaned her eyes with cotton balls and rubbed lotion on her skin to keep it hydrated. The fattest part of her leg was the same size as my little finger. Her skin was so transparent that I could actually see a hint of her inner organs working. I couldn't believe my eyes. The bililights, which were off at the time, were so strong that she'd developed quite a suntan. She opened her eyes and looked around several times. The nurses said that the eye muscles are very difficult to manage at this age. Her eyes were blue. She showed off quite a bit for us, and it was heartbreaking to leave her at 4 P.M. to go home for the first time in eleven days. Don was still at the wedding. Mom and Dad had to go home (a 225-mile drive), so I sat in my kitchen in the dark that night and cried. The stress of the last eleven days just had to come out.

Don and I went to the hospital together for the first time to see Sara when she was five days old. It was Father's Day, and sweet little

Sara had a card for her daddy. The bilirubin level was down to 4.6, her activity level was great, and her respiration was good. She went off the respirator at 6 P.M., and the transition to breathing on her own was hardly noticeable. She would still forget to breathe sometimes, but a tickle or a tap on her foot helped get her going again. I expressed milk for her before we left. Leaving that day was not as hard as the day before.

When I didn't go to the hospital, the nurses called me twice a day to report, once in the morning and again in the evening. Those calls were so important, and they were so nice to tell me things other than clinical, such as how she gave the nurses dirty looks when they were doing their checks on her or pricking her heel for blood samples. One night when she was given her every-half-hour dose of oxygen using a mask, her little face puckered up and she tried to cry. Nothing came out but a squeak because the respiration tube had irritated her throat. She turned red and got mad at everyone! She was slowly gaining weight but still hadn't reached her birth weight.

A schedule of visits soon developed with Don and me going together. Then I stayed for about four days of each week, and Don would go back to take care of the farm, return in four days, and take me home. I stayed at a rooming house across the street from the hospital. The owner told me that, amazingly, no matter when I came, there always seemed to be an empty room for me. Usually they were booked.

I was able to spend all day until about 8 P.M. with Sara. When she was ten days old, I got to hold her for the first time. The nurse put a preemie T-shirt on, which was big enough to go around her three times, and wrapped her up in a pink blanket. Disconnecting everything but the IV tubes, heart monitor, feeding tube, and oxygen, Sara was handed to me. I held the oxygen mask near her face while I held her for a very precious five minutes. It was the most wonderful experience of my new motherhood. She wiggled a little but never woke up. It had taken longer to get her ready to be held than the actual time spent holding her. I was grateful for the effort it took. The nurses said that she always behaved better when I was there. Everyone noticed that. Maybe they were trying to make me feel needed, I thought out loud. But, no, they were convinced that Sara knew when her family was visiting. It did make us feel good.

At twelve days old, Sara had an IV in her right ankle when her navel clotted over, a normal occurrence. Her tummy would distend, and all the feedings would have to stop. All she could have during this time was glucose and water. They watched her very closely during the night because a hole could develop in the intestine as a result of the distension. Her heart rate would drop, and so would her breathing. Still, the doctors said that this was not uncommon in preemie babies. One day when I was there, two-week-old Sara went into an apnea and bradycardia, a forget-to-breathe spell. Only one other nurse was in the room at the time, and she was feeding a full-term baby that had some feeding problems. I told the nurse that Sara had stopped breathing. The bells were going off on the heart monitor, and my heart rate was dropping right along with Sara's. I was told to tap her foot, which I knew how to do, but she wasn't coming out of it. She started turning gray, and I started yelling for the nurse to get over to her. Instead, she called a nurse from the hallway to come and hold the oxygen near her face. She obviously didn't know the procedure of putting the mask on her face to bag her. By this time Sara was as gray as a cement block. After about forty-five seconds of sheer panic on my part, Sara came out of it and started to breathe again. The doctor and two technicians came in and started working on her, taking more blood for tests. I was a wreck and started crying and couldn't stop. I went to the nursing room where I'd spent much time expressing milk for Sara. Her doctor came in and tried to comfort me, saying that her road was rocky but she was still doing very well. It was an awful day.

The next day, during morning rounds, I talked calmly and firmly to the full team of doctors about what had happened the day before. In the past I was often the only one in the room, briefly but alone. With four babies in that room all needing careful monitoring, I felt that things needed to change. Sara's doctor was shocked to hear about this, and within the hour things had changed. From then on, Sara and the baby next to her had a primary nurse. When that nurse came on duty, she would take care of those two babies only. When she went home, another nurse took on only those two. We were able to develop a trust. I often felt like a lioness guarding her young.

When Sara was four weeks of age and 1 pound 12 ounces, the IV in her ankle infiltrated and turned red. She was put on antibiotics to be on the safe side. She had been having more bradycardia spells and wasn't tolerating her feedings well. Her tummy would distend, feedings would stop, and she would lose weight again. Over and over she took one step forward and three steps backward. Her doctor mentioned the strong possibility of a surgical procedure to put in a TPN line, a larger IV inserted into the jugular vein in her neck that would travel to just above the heart. It would feed her high proteins, vitamins, and calories to force her over the hump of 1 pound 12 ounces. "She can't go home at one pound, twelve ounces," the doctor said. "We have to force her to grow." The thought of surgery for my tiny baby made me freeze, but I knew things had to improve quickly. We seemed to be getting nowhere.

We brought a crib mobile from home to put above Sara's bed. It revolved, and she seemed to enjoy the movement. A favorite music box of mine was also nearby. We wound it up, and she responded well to the sound. She looked around and wiggled as if she were dancing. Such a treasure. She was well rested and showing off. The respirator would build her energy level because it helped her breathe. Her ankle looked awful from the infiltrated IV site. It was black and crusty, and her leg was swollen. She was still on antibiotics to keep her safe from potential infection. Even though events seemed to be unpleasant, we were assured that Sara was doing well and took comfort in that. We were thankful for each new day because it meant another day closer to being home as a family.

After twenty-three days we were elated to find Sara in an isolette for the first time! She had graduated from the open bed to a more grown-up, less critical environment. Her doctor said that this round of feedings was her last chance to do well or the TPN line would be inserted. We prayed that she would respond favorably because the TPN line was one more potential infection site. Her weight was still at 1 pound 12 ounces. The antibiotics were discontinued, and her little ankle continued to heal, with a scar to remind us of her ordeal. Her oxygen was at 32 percent, and she was mostly breathing on her own. The apnea and bradycardia attacks still came frequently, but she seemed to come out of them a little easier. They were so worrisome.

The great day came at last when Sara finally passed her birth weight! She gained 30 grams and was now at 890 grams, slightly over 2 pounds. She was twenty-eight days old and measured one-half inch longer than at her birth. Her little cheeks looked pudgier, so that must have been where all her fat was going. Her doctor said that if people weren't hovering around her, she'd go into an apnea and bradycardia spell so they would come right over. He thought she was already spoiled and had all of them wrapped around her little finger. Was that possible for a wee little girl like that?

By day forty-eight, Sara had grown to 960 grams (2 pounds 2 ounces) but couldn't get over that hump. It was the same old story of tummy distension, backing off feedings, and losing weight. Her doctor said the next morning they would put in a TPN line. I was nervous but certainly willing to proceed. That night at the rooming house my first period after Sara's birth came. It was alarmingly heavy, and my stomach was very upset. Ironically, with all the medical facilities around, I called Don in the middle of the night and asked him to bring me to my own doctor at home. I felt like a horrible mother, abandoning my baby like that, but I was a hopeless wreck and ended up being a home for one week, fighting off fatigue and a low-grade fever. I was very grouchy about this ridiculous turn of events. The previous seven weeks must have taken their toll on me.

The TPN line was successfully inserted the next day, and that seemed to be the miracle boost Sara needed. She was put back on the open bed to make it easier for the nurses to care for her. From then on her weight gain was steady, the apnea and bradycardia attacks were fewer, and she maintained her body temperature. In one week she had gone from 960 to 1,090 grams, or 2 pounds 6½ ounces.

The TPN line stayed in until she was two months old for a total of twelve days. The line had caused her to look a little puffy. We were very hopeful that she would tolerate feedings now that the line was no longer feeding her. We had been blessed with a mom in the area who donated breast milk for her. I was unable to keep up with the stress and had dried up.

Finally, I was able to get back to the hospital and couldn't believe my eyes when I saw Sara. She had changed completely, to the point that I honestly wondered if she was truly our little Sara. The crib mobile was there as well as her ankle scar, so I figured she was indeed ours. She had gotten as fat as a 2-pound-6-ounce baby could get. She just looked huge, and we were overcome by all this.

Sara continued to have mild apnea and bradycardia spells but would come out of them with a tap to the foot. One time the nurse hollered at her, and she came out of it. Things began to improve daily, always with a few setbacks but generally in a positive direction. Weight gain was steady, and by day 65 she weighed 2 pounds 13 ounces. She had energy to show off and managed some acrobatics in the isolette, to which she had finally returned. Also, a big day came when she had clothes on for the first time.

Our time spent with her was now so much fun. She was acting more like a normal baby, looking around and even seeming to recognize us, or so we hoped. We could hold her for up to twenty minutes and took advantage of that time to start reading to her from a book about farm animals, of course. I gave her a bath for the first time, using a paper cup and a cotton ball. I sponged her all over and put lotion on her. She watched me ever so closely and grunted at me as we talked. I melted.

When Sara was ten weeks old, her charge nurse took me home to live with her when I was in town. I'd lost weight because my stomach had not been able to hold much since all of this began. Also, sleeping was elusive. The compassion she showed me was a blessing. As things improved at the hospital, I improved.

At eleven weeks, Sara's doctor really floored me. He said that Sara would be able to go home in about one week. She had graduated to a bassinet the week before, was handling herself well, and they called her a Neonatal All-Star. With the time I had spent helping care for her, he thought all would be well. As long as the coming week saw no setbacks, he expected her to be going home.

During rounds one day in her eleventh week, the eye specialist came to examine Sara. She was very cooperative until close to the end when she made sure he knew that she had had enough. The room was strangely quiet and tense. The doctor straightened up from the bassinet and, with a smile on his face, proclaimed Sara normal. A huge sigh of relief came from everyone in the room. They then informed me of the possibility of impairment or blindness as a result of prolonged oxygen exposure. I had never been told this, but that probably was for the best—one less thing to worry about. Needless to say, we all rejoiced together.

Sara's big day came at twelve weeks. She weighed 3 pounds 5 ounces, and she was going home. I had made her an eighteen-inch doll dress that she just swam in, but she looked precious. Her doctor said that she was probably the smallest baby from that unit to go home, and it was mainly because I had been there so much learning how to take care of her. It was pretty scary leaving the hospital. Everybody said they would miss her and wished us well. I thought we should take a nurse and a heart monitor with us, but that request wasn't necessary, they said.

Our first night home was a circus! Sara woke up for her 9 P.M. feeding and was awake and crabby until 3:30 A.M. Feeding, rocking, burping, singing, patting, and cuddling didn't seem to settle her down. Sara and I moved around the house and finally ended up in the living room. I turned on the lights, found the radio, and tried to duplicate the hospital environment. By this time my stomach was very upset, and I called her old room at the hospital. The nurse was concerned about me, not Sara. She knew Sara was okay but didn't know what to do about her wreck of a mom! Often Sara had been crabby at night and then would sleep it off. She was just being a baby, I was told. Don't worry.

We managed better after that first night. Both sets of grandparents helped a great deal, and I settled down to the daily and nightly routines of being a mom. Sara had to be awakened and fed every two hours around the clock. It would take an hour to feed her the necessary amount of formula, so sleep became a thing of the past. The grandmas helped with that, and soon we were all getting a bit more sleep.

We were told to keep all visitors away for a month except for grandparents. It was September, and the changing weather plus increased germ activity with schoolkids could be a threat to Sara's health. We were often showing our little bundle through the window to family and friends who stopped by to see our little miracle baby.

Sara's one-week checkup with her doctor left him amazed. She weighed 3 pounds 10 ounces and was 16¾ inches long. We had been told that once she got home, she would flourish. She proved that right and continued to grow steadily. The only potential problem we were warned about was that the scar on her ankle might cause problems as she got older. We were told that rubbing lotion on it, stretching the skin, and flexing the muscles would help. Otherwise, a plastic surgeon could do a graft to help give it more elasticity. It was possible that she wouldn't walk as easily because the scar might prevent her ankle from moving normally. We were committed to rubbing and stretching from that day on.

Sara's progress was positive but slow, it seemed. We learned quickly not to compare other one-year-olds to Sara because her experience was so unlike a full-term baby's. She sat up with help at one year and didn't talk until she was over three years old. We were patiently persistent and spent all our time doing the best we could in loving and nurturing. We were blessed with another baby girl when Sara was three years old. The cerclage was done at the proper time, and all went well with a 7-pound, full-term delivery. The two little sisters were the most precious gifts we could hope for.

Looking back on these events and recording them was a draining experience. All the emotions came flooding back, and I often had to wipe my eyes as the story unfolded. Sara is approaching her twenty-first birthday and has just completed her sophomore year in college. She is majoring in English because her flair for writing became evident as early as the first grade. Her teacher said then that she would be a writer one day. She has won writing contests through the years and even a $1,500 scholarship as a regional winner during the Iowa sesquicentennial.

Our miracle baby grew up as all kids do. She received a tremendous amount of help along the rocky road from people across the country we didn't even know who prayed for her. Her doctor once said that he was continually amazed by how babies so weak and tiny were literally willed by their parents to be strong and well. The power of prayer is an awesome thing, and we have living proof in Sara.

MARILYN'S DIARY: FIFTY-NINE DAYS IN THE NICU

by Stephanie and Dwight Dunbar

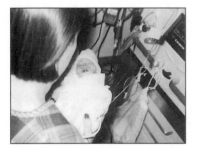
Marilyn, two days old.

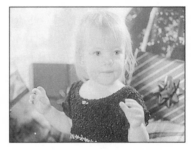
Marilyn, two years old.

I was shocked to find out I was pregnant last June. Now don't get me wrong; I really wanted to be pregnant, and I had just started taking Clomiphene to help me ovulate. When you are taking a drug like Clomiphene, you have to visit your doctor's office each month to have your blood checked to see if you ovulated. I was very excited to learn that my problem (not ovulating) could be easily fixed; however, I was equally disappointed to learn when I went in to get checked that I had not ovulated. My doctor had told me to call him when I started my period so he could write a prescription for more Clomiphene. I started having cramps around the normal time; they were the worst they had been in quite some time. After a week of not having actually started my period, other than a brief bout of spotting, I called the doctor's office to see if they would give me something to induce its onset. They said that would be fine but I would need to take a pregnancy test just to be sure.

So I diligently went to the store and bought a home pregnancy test. I decided not to take it that day; I was depressed enough because I had not ovulated while taking a drug that supposedly made ovulation happen. I didn't need it rubbed in by getting a negative result on a pregnancy test. The following morning I decided to get it over with. You cannot imagine my shock when I saw the little plus sign come up on the test. I wanted to believe it was true, but it couldn't be, could it? You can't get pregnant if you don't ovulate, and I didn't ovulate so I couldn't be pregnant. I decided there must have been something wrong with that particular test, so I went back to the store and bought a different brand. Once again the result was positive. I was elated; I really wanted this. Now I just had to hope that it wasn't some kind of cruel trick and that everything was as it should be.

I made an appointment to see my doctor and officially begin my pregnancy. They did all the usual things they do for people who have been taking fertility drugs. They did an ultrasound to make sure that the pregnancy was not a tubal one and to determine the number of fetuses. Once I was assured that everything was in the right place and that I was going to have only one baby, I went about the business of learning how to be pregnant. I bought books and read all about what was going on in my body, what I should be feeling, and the do's and don'ts of pregnancy.

My pregnancy progressed perfectly, according to my various resources. I was very fortunate not to get sick. I got pretty bad headaches for a few weeks but those went away, and I'll take just about anything over nausea. I was quite relieved to get through the first trimester safely and looked forward to the second trimester (when it's okay to look pregnant). My monthly checkups were fine. In October I had an ultrasound that indicated we were having a girl.

We decided to name her Marilyn Nicole. With four months to prepare for her arrival, we had not really started doing anything in terms of baby shopping or nursery preparation. We planned to begin all those things in November. Little did we know what was about to happen.

On November 11, I went to bed as usual. My husband, Dwight, stayed up late doing something on his computer. I awoke around 3:30 in the morning, which was not unusual; I often needed to get up and relieve myself in the middle of the night, especially as Marilyn was growing. (I am of the opinion that she knew exactly where my bladder was located and found it amusing to kick it and see how long it would take me to respond.) When I went back to bed, I was very uncomfortable. I recalled the pregnancy book mentioning that as the fetus gets larger, it may be difficult to get comfortable due to the pressure exerted on various organs when you are lying down. Following the book's advice, I changed my position to my side. No matter how I moved, I could not get comfortable. I was getting quite aggravated because I *never* have trouble sleeping, but in the back of my mind I thought that I should consider myself fortunate if this was my only pregnancy woe. After about twenty minutes of contemplating my dilemma, I noticed that my discomfort had turned into pain. I had no idea what to make of this, and while I was trying to figure it out, the pain turned into more pain.

Trying not to worry, I went downstairs and asked Dwight to be with me. When he asked why, I tried to explain that I was in pain, but I didn't really know how to explain the pain. He mistakenly thought I was just moaning and groaning about a tummy ache and didn't move to comfort me the way I had hoped. By the time I made it back to the bedroom, the pain had escalated and really alarmed me. I was scared because I had no idea what was happening, but I knew this kind of pain was not normal. I debated calling the doctor; it was 4:00 in the morning. I realize that most people wouldn't think twice about calling the doctor, but my father is a doctor, and he had frequently been woken up for something that could easily have waited or something he could do nothing about. I therefore thought I should evaluate my pain a little more thoroughly before deciding to wake my doctor.

By the time Dwight came upstairs, five minutes later, I was seriously considering what I should do. I was trying to read reference books about my problem, but every time I started reading, the pain would grip me just a little more and I couldn't concentrate on what the books said. Dwight kept asking me questions about what I was feeling, but I couldn't describe it. I couldn't figure out if I was going to be ill or if it was something else. Every time the pain got really bad and I could almost identify it, it went away and left me wondering if I had only a really bad stomachache. By this time it was almost 4:30 A.M. At Dwight's suggestion I called the doctor. She returned my call almost immediately and told me to come to the labor unit and let them take a look at what was going on.

I realize now that in the back of my mind I knew I was having contractions, but for some reason I would not let myself believe it. I was in my twenty-sixth week of the pregnancy. It was not possible for me to be having contractions. I had not had any problems; therefore, this could not be happening. I threw on some clothes and headed out to the car. I even stopped on the way out to get some work numbers so I could let them know I would not be in to work that day. I may have been in some sort of denial, but I did accept that something was wrong and that I would probably spend the day dealing with whatever that was.

By the time we left the subdivision, I was in the kind of pain that made my knuckles turn white from gripping the seats and kept me from talking. In between the pains I would talk to Dwight, who was amazingly calm. I can't remember what we talked about, but I am sure it concerned the pain and how I had not read anything about this kind of pain in my books. The hospital is only ten miles from our house, and at 4:45 in the morning the roads are virtually empty. Dwight was driving at an incredible speed, but still that trip to the hospital felt like an eternity.

As we turned onto the road that led to the hospital, my water broke. Once again I knew what had happened but could not bring myself to say it. I said something like "I just gushed stuff all over the seats of your truck." I must have been bordering on hysteria because I was thinking how amusing it was that Dwight wasn't upset about his car getting messed up (he's very particular about his cars). When we got to the hospital, we couldn't go to the labor unit because we didn't know where it was. The hospital tour was one of those things we were going to do sometime next month. Dwight pulled up to the emergency room entrance, and I was taken by wheelchair to the appropriate floor. I had gotten control of my near hysteria and achieved a state of calm with underlying fear. After all that stuff "gushed out," my pain lessened. I was convincing myself that they would check me out, make sure the baby was okay, give me some sort of medicine, and tell me to take it easy for a few days.

After I got into bed, the doctor explained to me what was happening—that my water had broken, but they would keep me in bed and try to delay labor. By the end of that sentence I just couldn't handle it anymore. I was sure she was going to say something about delaying labor, getting everything under control, and watching me closely for the rest of the pregnancy. Instead she said they would try to delay labor for about seventy-two hours and give me some drugs to help the baby's lungs mature. I think at this point I just tried to remove myself from my body. I couldn't have a baby yet. I was only twenty-six weeks pregnant. In the hysterical part of my mind that was starting to resurface, I remember thinking how only last week I had jokingly said, "Look, honey, it says here that if I have the baby now, they will be able to keep it alive." I didn't mean it; I certainly never considered it a possibility. I had never even given a thought to prematurity because I was having a healthy, no-problems pregnancy where I followed all of the "do's" and "don'ts." Premature babies are the result of some definite problem or too many drugs, right?

While trying to assimilate this concept of prematurity, I was also trying to pay attention to what the doctor was saying—that the baby was in a breech position and would probably need to be delivered by C-section. Now this might upset some people, but in the overall scheme of things I really didn't care anything about that because I still couldn't believe that in the next few days I would actually be having my baby, who was probably too immature to survive regardless of what those stupid books said. They never mentioned anything about any of this, now, did they? The doctor was saying that she just needed to check to see how dilated I was.

I was still trying to get a grip on what was happening when she said that she saw a foot and the umbilical cord. I was then informed that the baby was going to have to be delivered immediately. I appeared calm as she explained that there was no time for an epidural; they would have to put me out completely. I began to tune out. I focused on the sound of my baby's heart. Occasionally the baby would move, and they would lose the heartbeat. Each time I kept thinking they weren't going to get her out in time, but then they would move the monitor and her heartbeat would resume. I was trying not to panic, but it was obvious to me that the nurses were in quite a hurry. One nurse couldn't get my IV in and got so flustered that she jabbed the IV clear through to my vein and uttered a curse word. People were hovering over all parts of my body to prepare me for surgery. They were all telling me who they were and what they were doing. They put an oxygen mask over my mouth while I was trying to tell Dwight what numbers to call (once again, we didn't have a prepared list because we didn't think it was necessary yet).

When they started to wheel me to the operating room, I couldn't take it anymore and I began crying. I was sure Marilyn was not going to make it. All I could think about was how unfair life could be.

I had wanted this baby so badly. I had even waited until it was "safe" to start planning for her arrival. Now it was all going to be over. I prayed for everything to be the opposite of what I thought would happen, but I really didn't think anything could help at this point. Dwight walked beside me to the operating room and told me he loved me. I couldn't bring myself to tell him that we were about to lose our baby.

When I awoke, I was told that Marilyn was stable and that she was in the NICU. I can't even begin to describe how I felt. My baby was alive and was okay for the moment. I was excited, grateful, and terrified. She had made it into the world okay, but would she survive? As the first days passed, I began to believe that Marilyn would be all right. I probably could have just come out and asked, "Is she going to make it?" but I was afraid to hear the answer.

During our experience with the ups and downs of the NICU, Marilyn has always been stable and her problems minor compared to those of other preemies. I am very thankful that I have a beautiful baby girl. It wasn't very nice of her to come so early, and no one knows quite why she did, but I figure she must have had her reasons. After all, it's pretty hard to complain when your daughter is born on your birthday.

Marilyn's Diary: The NICU Chapter
11/12/96: DAY 1
Marilyn weighed in at 2 lbs. 3 oz., and was 14 inches long. Immediately after birth she was given Surfactant, a substance that helps maintain the expansion of the lungs to assure the transfer of oxygen throughout the body. Full-term babies and adults produce Surfactant, but premature babies lack this substance. She started off the day by being placed on a respirator, but by the end of the day she was breathing with the help of a CPAP (pronounced C-pap), continuous positive airway pressure. The CPAP helps her breathe by adding a little extra oxygen to what she breathes in. Marilyn's

"mommie" is doing great and hopefully will return home on 11/15/96. Unfortunately, little Marilyn won't be coming home to her new family until about February. God has really looked over her, and she is making great progress.

11/13/96: DAY 2

Nothing much happened today. She continues to breathe with the help of the CPAP. Her skin color is a little on the red side, and that is why she looks "sunburned" in the photo. She is undergoing phototherapy to control jaundice and gets to wear cool little sunglasses while the light is on.

11/14/96: DAY 3

Marilyn is moving right along in her little life. Today she got to come out of her incubator, and we held her for a few minutes. I heard her cry for the first time, and it was simply music to my ears. She has lost a little weight, but according to the doctor, that is to be expected.

11/15/96: DAY 4

Stephanie was released from the hospital today, and Marilyn lost a little more weight (1 lb. 14.5 oz). Marilyn was removed from the CPAP and placed on a nasal cannula. This just provides her with a little more oxygen than what she is getting from room air. It isn't easy for us to come home and leave her there, but we are looking forward to the day that she can come home. She had an ultrasound done on her head today to be sure there was no intracranial hemorrhaging. We are waiting to hear the news on that.

11/16/96: DAY 5

Today she was taken off the nasal cannula, and is breathing on her own. Right now she is experiencing a little bit of apnea, but the doctor doesn't seem very worried about it. The area of her brain that controls breathing is underdeveloped (as with all premature babies), and she forgets to breathe from time to time. A little stimulation will remind her to take a breath. She has lost a little more weight and now weighs at 1 lb. 13 oz. Her mommie got to hold her today while she slept. She was also taken off antibiotics, and her "mother's milk" was increased by .5 cc. We got the results from the ultrasound, and everything looks great. The doctors and we are really impressed by the amount of progress she is making.

11/17/96: DAY 6
Marilyn is still experiencing bouts of apnea and is receiving medication to help control it. Because blood has been taken from her to check for infections and to measure her oxygenation levels, she was given blood to replace what was taken. Her weight has come back up to 1 lb. 14 oz.

11/18/96: DAY 7
Today she had a rather severe bout of apnea while we were visiting, and the nurse had to rub her back to "remind" her to breathe. She was placed back on the nasal cannula supplying her with room air. This constant supply of air will help remind her to breathe. No change in weight.

11/19/96: DAY 8
Marilyn was placed on the CPAP today to help control the apnea and bradycardia that accompany it. She has gained a little more weight and now weighs 1 lb. 14.5 oz. She was a little jaundiced today, so the phototherapy was started again.

11/21/96: DAY 10
Marilyn is still breathing with the help of the CPAP. Her doses of aminophylline have been increased to help control the apnea and bradycardia. She gained 10 grams overnight, and the phototherapy

was stopped. She received another blood transfusion to help replace the blood that was taken for various tests. She has been on and off oxygen for the last two days. Oxygen has been around 22–23 percent. We got a chance to see the doctor's discharge plans, and he anticipates that she will be able to come home at thirty-six weeks of gestational age (about one month prior to her due date of February 16).

11/25/96: DAY 14

Not much happened these last few days. The doctor decided to remove Marilyn from the CPAP and place her on the nasal cannula, but that lasted only about three hours. Her apnea started up again, and they placed her back on the CPAP. She finally made it back to 2 lbs. today, and her mom and dad are so proud of her. She received another blood transfusion today. I am very grateful to our family, friends, and the students and staff of Dacula High School. Without their help, these last two weeks would have been much worse.

11/26/96: DAY 15

The nurses are starting to give the neonatologist a hard time about Marilyn being on the CPAP. Her little nose is getting sore from being on it, and the nurses want to give her a break from it. Marilyn's daddy went and gave blood today so that she would have some for the next transfusion. She gained an amazing 100 grams (3 oz.) and is now at 1,007 grams (2 lb. 4 oz.). The nurses couldn't believe the weight gain, so they weighed her three times to be sure. She was placed on a "bumper" bed today to help "remind" her to breathe. About every ten seconds Marilyn will be raised up a little and then sink back down. It is interesting to watch her going up and down in her incubator.

12/1/96: DAY 20

Things are progressing right along. Marilyn is still battling apnea and bradycardia, but they are now happening with less frequency.

She was off her CPAP for about an hour today and did real well without it. On 11/29/96 the NICU staff discovered that two of the babies had contracted the RSV virus. They were isolated from the rest of the others, but now we have to wear disposable gowns, gloves, and masks. I don't have much information on that particular virus, but I hope to find some soon. Her weight has been fluctuating a little, but right now she is holding at 1,045 grams (2 lbs. 5 oz.). I am so thankful to everyone who has included Marilyn in their prayers.

12/2/96: DAY 21
Today she was diagnosed with bronchopulmonary dysplasia (BPD), a condition of respirator-induced lung damage. She might also have NEC. The BPD, according to her doctor, seems to be mild. He intends to place her on steroids to help control it. This will also help end her apnea and bradycardia. Her doctor isn't sure about the NEC, but he feels it would be best to treat her for it with antibiotics just in case. It is fortunate if she does have NEC that it was found at an early stage. She now weighs 1,000 grams (2 lbs. 3oz.), and is 15½ inches long.

12/3/96: DAY 22
She was taken off the CPAP today and placed on the nasal cannula to give her nose a little rest. She seems to be doing well on it, and they might attempt to remove her from it if she continues to do well during the night. Her intake of breast milk has been stopped so that the doctor can deal with the NEC. She is receiving only IV fluids now and might be placed back on breast milk in seven days. She gained a little weight in the last twenty-four hours and weighs 1,035 grams (2 lbs. 4.5 oz.).

12/4/96: DAY 23
Well, she was placed back on the CPAP today. We got to see her little face for at least one visit. Treatment of the BPD will start once

the treatment for the NEC has stopped. Welcome aboard the NICU emotional roller coaster.

12/6/96: DAY 25
She was taken off her CPAP again today (it seems as though I have written that before). The NEC appears to be clearing up, and as a welcome side effect, so has the apnea and bradycardia. She continues to gain weight and now weighs 1,049 grams (2 lbs. 5 oz.).

12/9/96: DAY 28
Baby M has had a great couple of days. She has managed to stay off her CPAP and on a nasal cannula. Weight has increased every day, and she now weighs 1,134 grams (2 lbs. 8 oz.). She was given an extra dose of aminophylline to help control the apnea and bradycardia. Her feedings of breast milk were started again today, and she is receiving 1 cc/hour. Her length was measured last night, and she is now 15¾ inches long. Her antibiotic treatments for the NEC will stop tomorrow. She is receiving 26 percent oxygen through her nasal cannula.

12/11/96: DAY 30
She was placed back on the CPAP on 12/9/96 because her apnea and bradycardia were happening more frequently. She continues to gain weight and now weighs 2 lbs. 10.2 oz. The NEC seems to be well under control. Nothing much else has happened the last few days.

12/12/96: DAY 31
Happy Birthday.

12/13/96: DAY 32
Breast milk intake increased to 2 cc/hr. She is still on her CPAP but is able to take a break from it when we come to visit. She is breath-

ing room air, but occasionally she is given additional oxygen. Stephanie got to hold her for over two hours skin to skin, but she became a little tired and began to have spells of apnea and bradycardia. She receives her milk by gavage feeding. The doctor is waiting to increase her breast milk until she stools again.

12/14/96: DAY 33

I got to hold her for a little while today. She wasn't wearing her CPAP, so we were able to give her the aerosol treatment. She seems to enjoy the treatment because she smiles a little while getting it. We were able to stay while the nurses weighed her. She becomes real active during weighing, kicking and swinging her little arms. She now weighs 1,265 grams (2 lbs. 13 oz.).

12/15/96: DAY 34

Today was a big day for all three of us. She was taken off the CPAP and placed on the nasal cannula. (We think this is because she likes her weekend nurse). This may not last long, but we will have to wait and see. We arrived in the NICU just in time to participate in giving her a bath and weighing her. Stephanie bathed her while I videotaped it all. We hadn't realized how dependent we have become on her various monitors until tonight. While Marilyn was being bathed and weighed, her monitors were disconnected. She did fine while off the monitors, but we felt as if a big weight were lifted from us when she was reconnected. Marilyn's grandmother and great-grandmother came to see her, and her grandmother got to hold her for a little while. She is still receiving 2 cc/hr of breast milk, 6 cc/hr of IV fluids, and .5 cc/hr of intralipids. I told you it was a big day.

12/17/96: DAY 36

Wow. Another surprise. She was taken off her nasal cannula this morning and has gone all day with no episodes of apnea or bradycardia. We decided to visit her later at night so that we could help to bathe and weigh her. Being able to participate in her "activities" makes us feel a little more like parents. She had her eye appointment today, and I am happy that everything looks normal. There are so many things to be afraid of, but thankfully we can put ROP at the bottom of that list. Her breast milk was increased to 2.5 cc/hr at full strength. (It was a 50-50 solution of water and breast milk). Oh, yeah, she topped 3 lbs. today. She weighed in at 1,396 grams (3 lbs. 1 oz.). I wonder what tomorrow will bring.

12/18/96: DAY 37
Still going strong without the nasal cannula or CPAP. She had only one spell of apnea and bradycardia today, and that is down from the usual five per day she was having last week. She continues to gain weight and is 1,431 grams (3 lbs. 2.5 oz.). Her breast milk was increased to 3 cc/hr, the IV was dropped to 5 cc/hr, and the intralipids are at .7 cc/hr. I finally felt comfortable enough to give her a kiss tonight, and a big smile came across her face. It probably was only a random facial expression, but it still made me feel good.

12/20/96: DAY 39
Pretty much the same. Weight is now 1,492 grams (3 lbs. 4.5 oz.), breast milk at 3.5 cc/hr, intralipids at .7 cc/hr, and IV fluids at 5 cc/hr.

12/23/96: DAY 42
Marilyn had a great weekend. Her grandmother and great-grandmother came to see her again, and both were able to hold her. She is doing very well on her feedings and has been changed from a continuous feeding to a scheduled feeding. She receives 12 cc every three hours. She isn't big enough to bottle-feed; she doesn't have the sucking, swallowing, breathing reflex perfected yet. She is on a larger size pacifier, and she gets to suck on the pacifier while receiv-

ing her feeding. This helps her associate nursing with a full tummy. The NICU staff will attempt bottle feeding in about three days, and if that goes well, they anticipate being able to remove her IVs. She has really grown a lot over this past week. She is now 16¼ inches long and weighs 1,616 grams (3 lbs. 9 oz.). The apnea and bradycardia have almost completely stopped. She has a spell only once in about twenty-four hours. Her doctor told us that one day she would just stop. All her little NICU friends are going home, and what started out to be a full NICU will be down to two babies by tomorrow. That will make Marilyn the "senior" NICU baby.

12/24/96: DAY 43

We received a great surprise today when we went to visit Marilyn. One of the nurses decided that since she was awake and alert, she would try to bottle-feed her, and she did great with it. We went back for her next feeding, and she did it again. Needless to say we were completely surprised since the NICU staff thought that it would be another week or so before she would be able to bottle-feed. We couldn't have asked for a nicer Christmas present from her. We were still at the hospital when Santa arrived at 2 A.M. on the 25th. Marilyn wasn't too interested in seeing Santa, so Santa filled her stockings with toys and cards from the family.

12/25/96: DAY 44

She is still doing great with the bottle, and her doctor wants us to bottle-feed her once a day. The others are gavage feedings. Gavaging consists of feeding Marilyn through a tube that runs from her nose to her stomach. They will increase her intake of breast milk by 1 cc every twelve hours (currently she is getting 15 cc/feeding). She isn't doing too well with her IVs because she keeps pulling them out, so the NICU staff hopes to wean her from them in three or four days. When we arrived at the NICU for her 7 P.M. feeding, we found a Christmas card from her waiting for us. I wondered what she did with all her spare time, and now I know. Her weight is now at 1,673 grams (3 lbs. 11 oz.).

12/26/96: DAY 45

The other baby that was in the NICU with Marilyn died today. He was a twenty-five-week preemie and had a severe case of BPD. It forced us to reflect on the past six weeks and realize just how fortunate we really are. Marilyn had a few problems, but nothing like her NICU friend. My thoughts and prayers will continue to go out to his family.

12/28/96: DAY 47

Marilyn is doing well with her bottle, and the nurses are trying to feed her from the bottle every three hours. Right now she can only bottle-feed well three times a day, while the rest of the time she is gavage-fed. Marilyn is running out of IV spots, so the doctor told the nurses not to reinsert another once this IV goes bad. Well, she is now off the IV and is receiving all her nourishment from the bottle. They are also turning down the temperature in her incubator in an attempt to move her into a bassinet. This means she will probably not gain weight as fast as she has because she will be expending additional calories keeping warm. It looks as if we are getting close to her coming home.

12/30/96: DAY 49

I got a chance to speak with her doctor today, and he anticipates her coming home in about seven to ten days. It is so hard to believe that she might be home that soon, but before she comes home she must be able to maintain her body temperature while sleeping in a bassinet and also be able to take all her feedings from the bottle. Right now she is still sleeping in an incubator, but the temperature continues to drop a little each day. She weighed in last night at 4 lbs. 1 oz., and we are so proud of her.

1/9/97: DAY 59

The day has finally arrived, and little Marilyn is heading home. We never would have thought that after spending fifty-nine days in the NICU she would be coming home almost six weeks before her due date. She came home on an apnea monitor and is taking medication to help prevent any apnea. She now weighs 4 lbs. 10 oz. and is 16¾ inches long. What a change from the 2 lbs. 3 oz. little girl I first met on November 12. I guess this closes the NICU chapter of her life and opens an entire book of experiences to come.

THE LITTLE BATTLER: TRACE'S STORY

by Michelle Rhames

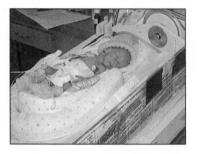

Trace, six weeks old, 1 pound 12 ounces.

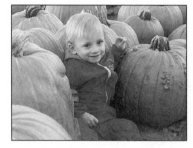

Trace, nineteen months old.

My husband and I loved the name Trace the first time we heard it, and we knew if we ever had a son that Trace would be his name. Years later we found out the name had an Irish derivation that meant "battler," but it wasn't until our baby had to fight for his life that we fully realized how perfect this name was. I truly believe we were chosen, perhaps long ago, to be this special child's parents. It has been the hardest but also the best thing we have ever done.

We were a bit surprised but so happy when we learned during a routine checkup that I was pregnant. I had been off birth control (by choice) for only a few weeks, and we had expected it to take about a year for my system to readjust and allow conception. Right away we purchased a rocking chair, and I took excellent care of myself. However, it didn't take long for complications to arise. The first problem I had was spotting and bleeding during the first trimester. I felt sure I would miscarry, and one day I sat in the bathroom and cried as blood dripped steadily from my body. We drove to the ER, which was an hour away on the snowy Idaho highway, but we were reassured that the cervix was closed and that I should just rest until we could see the OB-GYN and have an ultrasound. That weekend I quit my part-time job and started modified bed rest, which only allowed me to get out of bed to use the bathroom and shower. Monday we went to see the doctor, and an ultrasound confirmed that our baby was doing very well. The tiny being inside me was doing flips and waving its arms. My husband and I were so relieved and excited. Just before we left the office that day the doctor suggested I take a triple marker screening test for Down's syndrome and spinal anomalies. It was a simple blood test, so I agreed.

A few days later we were shocked when the doctor called and told me I needed to come in immediately. The test had come back positive for a spinal abnormality. He said it was probably a false positive and that it happened all the time. The test screened for spina bifida and other serious defects, so we were very scared. The doctor suggested a higher-level ultrasound to check the baby's spine, and maybe amniocentesis. Since my husband is in the Air Force we were flown two states away to Washington in order to go to a military facility that could administer the testing. I vividly remember the week because I had just started to feel the baby kicking. The ultrasound was done on Valentine's Day and showed that our baby was a boy. The doctor in Washington said that he was 98 percent certain our son had no spinal abnormality but casually mentioned that in his experience mothers who had positive results on this test often had other complications such as premature babies and that I needed to see my doctor more often. We left there with huge smiles on our faces and called our family from the lobby. We were going to have a son, and he did not have a spinal defect! We thought the worst was behind us. We had no idea that this was only the beginning.

My husband was deployed to Saudi Arabia near the end of my fifth month of pregnancy. Our baby was due June 30, and my husband was scheduled to be back barely two weeks before then. I had just begun to show a small round belly, and I was devastated that he would miss my entire third trimester. I had no idea then that even I would miss my third trimester! I cried my heart out when he left. I had made plans to visit my family in Florida for a few weeks right after my husband was deployed so that my mother could pamper me and lift my spirits. I packed a bag of maternity gear and left on March 7. I never got to wear the maternity clothes, and I never returned to our home in Idaho. One should never plan things too rigidly because life has its own plan sometimes.

The day my plane landed in Florida my feet swelled up like hams. I had had a long day of travel and a serious altitude and weather change, so I didn't give it a second thought. Right before I left Idaho, I had gone to the doctor, and everything was normal except for a trace amount of protein in my urine. The doctor suspected a urinary tract infection and told me to drink some cranberry juice and to have a nice time in Florida. I now know that the protein and swelling were signs of early preeclampsia, but at the time I had no idea. That first week I kept bloating more and more, and then the headaches began. I attributed these to normal pregnancy discomforts. The next week the bloating was up to my knees, and I was drinking fluids but urinating less and less. The most alarming development was that my baby's movements were lessening, and eventually there was no movement at all. I had brought my pregnancy guidebook to read, and I started to suspect preeclampsia but figured I was just a paranoid pregnant woman. I felt different, but I didn't feel *sick*. Nevertheless, we decided to go to my mother's OB-GYN for peace of mind. When the doctor examined me, I was very relieved to hear the baby's heartbeat. I was twenty-five weeks along in the pregnancy. They checked my blood pressure, but the nurse felt sure she had done something wrong because of the high reading. The next reading was even higher. They did a urine test and checked my reflexes, which were very brisk. The doctor left the room and didn't come back for what felt like hours. When he did come back, he said I was in severe kidney failure and in the advanced stages of preeclampsia. I needed to go to the emergency room immediately. I started to cry, and my mother held me as they tried to explain this disease to me. I didn't hear or understand too much of what he said because I was so upset.

We went straight to the hospital, which was only two minutes from the doctor's office. I was immediately put on magnesium sulfate to control seizures. They also inserted a Foley catheter, which drained my bladder around the clock and let them monitor my kidneys. That night the kidney specialist assessed my condition and recommended we deliver the baby right away because this was the only way to stop the progression of this disease, which could leave me with permanent kidney damage or worse. I had no idea what this meant. I believed that my baby would come out small but perfect. I didn't even know that Neonatal Intensive Care Units existed.

The Red Cross began the long process of getting my husband home from Saudi Arabia for emergency leave. The perinatologists wanted to wait as long as we could to deliver the baby. They administered antenatal steroids to help the baby's lungs mature. The next day an ambulance transported me to the large city hospital downtown that had a level IV NICU. My kidneys began to improve, and then worsened. My husband arrived on my fourth day in the hospital. He sat by my side every minute as the nurses emptied my catheter bags, which were now sometimes purple from all the blood in my urine. We kept waiting to give the baby more time to develop in the womb. On the sixth day blood tests showed that my liver was not functioning properly. HELLP (hemolysis, elevated liver enzymes, and low blood platelets) syndrome was confirmed on the seventh day, and an emergency cesarean section was performed. HELLP syndrome is a serious disease that is very rare and causes liver failure. The damaged liver cannot produce enough platelets to maintain blood clotting, so the mother can bleed to death. Delivering the baby quickly was the only option to save my life.

That first night was so difficult. My husband was told that I was transported to the cardiac ICU while our baby boy went to the NICU. Our twenty-six-weeker son weighed only 1 pound 7 ounces (660 grams) at birth. He had to be intubated and put on a respirator right away because he could not breathe on his own. They gave my husband little hope for the baby or his wife. The complicated delivery had been under general anesthesia, so my husband and I did not witness the birth. My husband got his first swift glance at our son as they wheeled the incubator to the NICU, and I didn't get to see the baby for three days. I spent a couple of days in the cardiac ICU, but my condition improved dramatically once the baby was delivered. I was transferred to the regular postpartum ward to recover. They told us that the baby's first few days would be crucial; if he survived the first few days, his chances for making it would drastically improve. My first look at the baby was not what I expected: They brought a Polaroid picture to the ICU so I could see him. His skin was charred looking, and there were tubes in his mouth and tape all over his face. The photo showed only his face and a bit of his upper torso. The picture didn't show how tiny he really was. My first NICU visit was my reality check.

The NICU was on the fourth floor of the hospital, while the regular maternity ward was on the third. It was very reassuring to know that the baby was so close, and I could visit him around the clock. My husband took me to the NICU in a wheelchair as soon as I could get out of bed. I must admit I was scared to visit Trace. I didn't know what to expect and was afraid to love such a frail baby. Soon I realized that I had loved him from the moment I knew he was inside me and that it was no use trying to guard against the possible hurt I might feel if he died. Besides, I was his mother, and he needed me.

The first time I saw Trace I could only see his tiny hand and arm because he was wrapped tightly in blankets. His entire hand was the size of my thumbnail, and later I saw that his leg was the width of my pinkie. He had so many tubes and wires going into his tiny body that he didn't look at all like a baby. The worst thing—the thing I will never forget—is the way his chest went up and down with the rhythm of the ventilator. He appeared to have no real life of his own. He was being kept alive with many machines, and I just cried when I imagined his immense suffering beneath all those needles, tubes, and bright lights. He had an IV in both arms and behind one of those tiny legs. I wanted to leave right away that first visit. We went to visit every day, a few times each day. Friends brought us a book about premature babies, and we made Trace an audiotape of our voices reading *Stuart Little* so that the nurses could play it for him when we couldn't be there.

I had some complications with the healing of my abdomen and with an esophageal tear from surgery. The doctors had to cut through layers of scar tissue in order to get the baby out, and I lost lots of blood due to HELLP syndrome. I was discharged a week after the delivery and then returned as an outpatient for wound care for three weeks. I felt so empty the day I was discharged. I thought it would be wonderful to finally get out of the hospital, but it was a nightmare because I felt so far away from our baby. The day I left I saw a woman being wheeled out with her full-term baby. I wondered if I would ever get the chance to take my son home, and at the same time I was glad that I still had a son at all.

Trace was the smallest baby in the NICU, and the sickest at the time. The list of drugs by the isolette was at least ten names long. He immediately developed PDA. The open ductus of the heart that nourishes the lungs with blood in the womb closes automatically at a term birth. In preemie babies the ductus often remains open and complicates the respiratory distress they already have from pulmonary insufficiency because the blood keeps flooding the lungs. A drug called indomethacin closed it within a few days. If the drug hadn't worked, surgery would have been necessary to close the ductus. We had overcome one of the many NICU obstacles.

That first month Trace developed lots of complications, and we could never be certain that he would make it. The hardest part was watching him endure so many painful medical procedures. Right after the delivery they discovered a bilateral IVH—a brain bleed on both sides of his head. They range in severity from a grade one (least severe) through four. Trace had a grade two that never progressed any further. I will never forget one set of parents we met in the hospital support group. Their little girl was born a few weeks after Trace, so we passed each other in the halls on our daily visits or at the sinks as we scrubbed before seeing the babies. Their daughter was hanging on, and then she suddenly developed a grade four bleed. I had read about the IVH risks and knew this was not good news. Within two days her isolette was gone, and although the staff was very discreet about patient information, I knew their daughter had died because I never saw the parents again. The night I realized their daughter had died I called the NICU nonstop to check on Trace. The nurses were always so wonderful and talked me through tough times like these. They were the only link I had to my son on those long nights when we didn't know if he was improving or not. The phone became so important because they had reassured us they would call if his condition worsened at all. Every time it rang that first month, our hearts would stop for a moment in terror.

Trace was on steroids to help his lungs mature so that the staff could wean him off the ventilator. These steroids made his blood sugar unstable, so he had to have insulin to control it. This meant he had to have heel sticks every few hours to check his blood sugar. His heels were constantly purple and bandaged. He also had trouble with jaundice, and he was placed under the bilirubin lights on and off for a while. His iron levels were always low, so they had to give him four blood transfusions and a drug called Erythropoetin for eighty-five days. Trace needed IVs for nutritional support and many medications. Eventually preemies have their heads shaved and IVs inserted in their scalps when the veins in their arms and legs break down. It doesn't take long for a preemie to run out of usable veins. Within a few weeks I was approached to sign a consent form for a central vein line (CVL). The doctors did not anticipate that Trace would be off IV support for months. The CVL meant that he would have a larger line inserted surgically into a large access near the heart. There would be an exit incision on his neck. I agonized over this decision, but after the procedure Trace's morale really improved. He could now have all his IV fluids, medications, and blood transfusions fed into this line. I could sense that he was happy with the decision and felt more comfortable, although I hadn't even held him yet.

Probably the most trying hurdle for any micropreemie is respiratory trouble. They are born with tiny immature lungs that usually are not capable of breathing on their own. The ventilator breathes for the baby or just helps him breathe, and every preemie has his own unique struggle weaning from this machinery. The vent can work aggressively for the weakest preemies, and gently for the stronger ones—through frequency of breaths and percentage of oxygen. These two numbers were the first things we asked every time we saw our son. A monitor reads the oxygen saturation in the baby's blood, and the vent is set accordingly. The vent can be set as high as 100 percent oxygen, but the lower the setting, the better. Forcing oxygen into preemie lungs causes serious problems. One danger is the possibility of collapsing the fragile lungs, and another is creating permanent scar tissue. However, there are risks inherent to not giving the baby enough oxygen—such as brain damage. We fought the oxygen battle for six weeks. After that he was able to go to a CPAP machine—continuous positive airway pressure. He was taken off the

CPAP within a few days, but he was constantly watched for apnea (when the baby stops breathing) to be sure he was ready to breathe by himself. When he was finally free of all respiratory support, we were at last able to hold him. It was a wonderful, magical time since this was also the first time I could see Trace's face without tape or tubes.

The first time I held Trace it was for only a few minutes, and I was so surprised by how light he was. At the time he only weighed 1 pound 12 ounces, so it felt as if I was holding an empty blanket. I held him first, and then I let my husband have extra time holding him because only days later my husband had to return to work in Idaho. The military had let him have two months, and it was time to go back. We both cried because we knew he wouldn't be able to fly out again until the baby was discharged, which could still be months away.

Another huge obstacle for preemies is nutrition. At birth Trace's digestive system was too immature to sustain breast milk or formula. He had to be given IV nutrition exclusively for many weeks. Slowly, they tried to give him minuscule amounts of breast milk, which I had pumped for him. Pumping breast milk was the one thing only I could do for my son, which was why it was important to me. Yet my milk never came in appropriately, so pumping was a long, sometimes painful process. The nurses explained that my body may have been too stressed or busy healing to facilitate a steady flow of milk. I also mourned the normal bonding I should have had with my baby as I sat pumping the milk with the huge, cold pump. Trace would sometimes tolerate the milk, but too often his abdomen would become distended and we would have to stop the feeds and go back to the IV. This happened to us many, many times, which was scary because each time his stomach swelled the doctors put him on antibiotics and warned us about NEC. Necrotizing enterocolitis is a very serious complication that affects portions of the baby's intestines. Sometimes these infected sections die and must be surgically removed. Trace never developed full-blown NEC, but he had many NEC scares, and too many times we prayed our hearts out by his isolette waiting for a bowel movement. A healthy bowel movement meant so much to us then. We would celebrate when they came because they meant that his intestines were functioning.

Trace gained weight very slowly. While other babies were moving to the back of the nursery where the healthier babies were transported, Trace remained in the critical care section. Sometimes days would go by with either weight loss or no change in weight. Since the babies had to meet weight and wellness guidelines for discharge, I felt sure we would never get to leave the NICU. By the third month in the NICU, Trace started to progress. It was very slow, but he did get better each day and even started to gain some weight. His primary nurse was an advocate of kangaroo care; this is when the baby is placed skin to skin with their parents. The numbers on Trace's monitors were very high during these sessions, which indicated that he was benefiting from this therapy. One by one the machine and pumps were wheeled away from his bedside.

Unlike full-term children, who know how to suckle at the breast or bottle at birth, preemies need to be taught how to do this. The lessons were hard work for Trace. Often babies start to have frequent apnea spells during feeds, and they get exhausted after only a few minutes. He gained at half the normal rate, but he was steadily gaining and managed to stay fairly healthy. A cold or other illness in the NICU environment can be deadly to a fragile preemie. Their immune systems are simply not ready to fight off diseases or get well without complications. Trace was repeatedly tested for sepsis because they suspected his slow progress was caused by this blood disease. It was always ruled out.

The last two months in the NICU I spent almost the entire day at the hospital. Sometimes I would be there for eight to ten hours straight because he was finally strong enough for me to cuddle for longer stints, and the nurses would save his bath time for me. Since he was such a slow gainer, they tried to keep him in his bed resting as much as possible. I was also able to give him occasional bottles, although he usually alternated bottle feedings with gavage feedings. Gavage feedings are given through a tube inserted in the baby's nose or mouth that goes directly to the stomach. Trace had a permanent gavage tube for many weeks. At this time I was also able to buy him tiny preemie clothing and dress him. It was only in the last two months that I had a few family members and close friends come to visit him. This was when we started to actually dream and hope for a future.

For Trace's final month he was transferred to the back of the nursery. This was a huge triumph for us because it meant we were on our way home. The nurses had to make sure I knew how to give him his feedings, baths, and basic care. The monitors indicated that Trace was greatly improving since he stopped having apnea spells and bradycardia spells, which was encouraging for us. The doctors checked him constantly for an inguinal hernia because he had developed a hydrocele, a small opening that usually develops into a hernia. Also, his eyes were checked for retinopathy of prematurity. This is when abnormal blood vessels and scar tissue grow over the retina, a problem that can cause blindness if not treated. Trace developed a mild case of retinopathy, but he did not need the usual laser eye surgery before discharge. His hydrocele healed itself, and when Trace reached 4 pounds 8 ounces, we were finally able to bring him home. Trace had been at the NICU for so long that I knew he would be missed by the nurses, doctors, and staff who had cared for him so well. Before we went home I decorated the nurse's lounge with party supplies and brought in various pastries to thank them for being so wonderful to our son and our family. We were finally on our way home!

Home had been changed because Idaho lacked the adequate follow-up care for Trace. The military moved us to Virginia, and after Trace's discharge, my husband came to pick us up and we were finally a family again. When we first brought Trace home we put him in a basinette in our bedroom. Trace was discharged with no monitors or supplemental oxygen because he was doing so well. Still, we panicked about every move he made, and we were terrified that he would stop breathing at night and we wouldn't know it. Trace had some minor reflux problems, which meant that he vomited almost everything we fed him. When he first came home, it took almost two hours to feed him because his sucking was so weak. I started to feed him bottles and formula because my milk supply had dwindled to nothing. We had to prop him up in the bed with pillows to help him digest his meals. The first few months were tough, but we were so happy to have him home at last that we handled it well. We kept him in total isolation to prevent his getting sick and having to return to the hospital. I sterilized everything he touched and sanitized the house constantly. I had planned on being a stay-at-home mom for at least a couple of years, and this became a necessity because Trace needed some time for his lungs to heal. Using the ventilator had left some minor scarring on his lungs, so the doctors urged us to do our best to keep him from getting sick for at least two years.

It has been almost one year since our baby was discharged from the hospital. He has had his first birthday and has been sick only twice. At discharge they stressed the importance of physical and developmental follow-ups. At the time we didn't know that we would be seeing so many doctors and what they would be preparing us for, but now we do. Trace has some minor delays in gross motor skills, speech, and fine motor skills. We cannot be sure if he is just catching up from an early birth and a traumatic beginning in life or if he has some brain damage from the brain bleeds and other complications. For the delays he receives physical therapy, occupational therapy, and speech therapy every week. The therapists come to our home to keep him from getting sick. We take him to the pediatric ophthalmologist to check the progression of his ROP. It has resolved but has left Trace very nearsighted. He will definitely wear glasses by the time he goes to kindergarten.

Our biggest concern today is for his future and what it will be like. We prepare for the worst and hope for the best. Some days we can't believe we have been so blessed, and some nights we cry because we know that his life will be full of special challenges. Right now he is a happy baby who crawls everywhere, pulls up on furniture to stand, and smiles at everyone, enchanting them with his huge blue eyes. At fifteen months he weighs only 16 pounds, but he is very muscular and can climb every stairway in our home. Most of all he swells our hearts with joy and fills our home with sweet laughter, and we cannot imagine our life without him in it.

GUARDED BY ANGELS . . .
FOREVER AN ANGEL

by Susie Bakken-Lang

My story is an unusual one because it is about my father and not my child. On December 9, 1921, my father, Orvin Bakken, was born on a farm in northeast Iowa. According to my grandma, he came into the world quite suddenly and was not due until the "early part of March." Dad weighed in at 1 pound 4 ounces. He was very tiny and could easily fit in the palm of my grandpa's hand. Dad's arms were so small that Grandpa's wedding ring could go all the way to his shoulder and still have room to spare.

My grandma had a strong faith in God, and she knew her first-born son would need more than just her to watch over him. On December 10, 1921, Dad was baptized. Grandma knew he was now truly a child of God and in God's care.

What I have to tell you next may seem hard to believe, but if you will stop for a minute and remember that seventy-seven years ago there were no NICUs, no incubators, and no specialized nursing, you will understand that what Grandma did was necessary to keep her child alive. With limited resources Grandma had three things to rely on: creativity, common sense, and prayer.

In the kitchen of the farmhouse there was a wood-burning stove, and connected to it was an oven. By keeping enough wood in the stove to heat the oven, the oven maintained enough heat to keep Dad warm without creating a fire hazard. Dad's incubator was actually a shoe box that once was home to a pair of Grandpa's shoes. This was Dad's bed for the rest of the winter.

With no apnea monitors or IVs my grandma's greatest concerns were his breathing, whether he was getting enough to eat, and whether he was maintaining his body temperature. The only technology she could rely on was her lifeline to God through prayer.

I remember Grandma telling me and my cousin about Dad being so small that he didn't know how to suck from her, so she would take a small dropper, put a couple of drops of milk in his mouth, and then rub his tiny throat so he would swallow. When he grew a little bigger, she would put the breast milk on a small spoon and feed him. In time he was strong enough to nurse.

With all that Dad had going against him, he never had any physical or mental handicaps. He was very seldom sick but did have surgery on his stomach and colon at the age of forty-four. He recovered fully from his surgery and never had any recurring problems. When Dad passed away at age sixty-nine, he still had his tonsils.

Even though Dad was born early and was small, he was a very intelligent man. He wore the hats of businessman, veterinarian, accountant, mechanic, and carpenter. After all, he was a successful farmer. His lifelong partner, my mom, and their six children were always amazed at how fast he could do math in his head and not use a pen and paper. He had a great sense of humor and a heart as big as the great outdoors. He was a kind, gentle man, all five feet one inch of him!

MEGAN: OUR SWEET BABY GIRL

by Nancy Lynn Redheffer

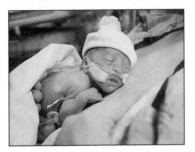

Megan, five days old, kangarooing with her dad.

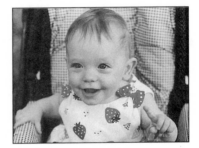

Megan's first birthday.

Our baby girl was born on our second wedding anniversary. At twenty-seven weeks and six days of gestational age, Megan Elizabeth weighed 1,145 grams or 2 pounds 8 ounces, and measured 15 inches in length. Three days before Megan's birth I noted that I was feeling less fetal movement. The following evening I experienced blood spotting. After an examination by my obstetrician, several hours on a fetal monitor, and an ultrasound, I was sent home. Everything appeared to be fine. The afternoon before Megan's birth I began to experience what felt like menstrual cramps that became increasingly worse. I returned to the hospital and spent several hours on a fetal monitor before the doctor determined I was having contractions. A pelvic exam revealed that my cervix was dilated 1 centimeter. Magnesium sulfate was administered in an unsuccessful attempt to

stop my preterm labor, and I received a dose of the steroid betamethasone to accelerate the baby's lung development.

Until that point my husband, David, and I both naively believed
that my labor would be stopped and that although I might need to
spend a day or two in the hospital, everything would be fine. Yet the
cramps, as I still thought of them, worsened. I felt increasing pressure on my pelvic floor—the baby's head. Suddenly I was dilated 8 or
9 centimeters. I was told the baby was coming *now!* The next thirty
minutes were horrific. David and I were terrified. It was much too
soon for our baby to come. How could she survive?

After her birth I asked over and over again if my baby would be
all right, but no one answered. I pleaded with them to help her. She
was intubated, stabilized, and taken to the Special Care Nursery. I
never saw her in the birthing room. David later told me that she was
blue and was not breathing. I felt so empty. I was not pregnant anymore, yet I did not have my baby.

Over the next hour the obstetrician, the neonatologist, and the
special care parent liaison each visited with us. They were very kind
and supportive, as they would be for the months to come. They explained what was happening and offered realistic projections for her
survival and recovery. We were told that we were welcome in the
nursery twenty-four hours a day. We were given Polaroid photographs of our baby girl. I later learned that the photos were de-
ceiving because the tubes attached to our baby were as scaled down
in size as she was. Yet the photos were a great comfort. Her head was
rather bruised, but she looked better than I had imagined.

David went to the nursery to see our baby. When he returned to
me, he was crying. I had never seen him so afraid. We decided to
choose a name for her before we went to the nursery together.
Ironically, weeks earlier we had planned to choose a name on that
very day, our wedding anniversary. On my way from the birthing
center to the maternity ward, I was taken into the nursery to see
Megan. She looked much worse in person. She was so thin and red,

and there were so many tubes, wires, and machines attached to her. I could not imagine that it was possible for her to survive.

Once I saw her, the feelings of guilt were overwhelming. I remember thinking over and over again, *she doesn't deserve this.* Despite numerous tests, the cause of my preterm labor was never determined. I asked what I had done wrong. My doctor reassured me that it was probably not caused by something I had control over, but I felt completely responsible nevertheless. My baby girl was suffering so much, and I could not help her. Also, I felt horribly cheated. I missed virtually the entire third trimester of my pregnancy. We saw other couples in the maternity ward who were beaming with happiness. Other rooms were filled with flowers, balloons, happy visitors, and healthy babies. Our family and friends were understandably horrified when they heard the news. It didn't feel like a time for celebration. Yet we were also very grateful. Not a moment went by in the first days that I didn't think about how close to death our baby was and that we were so very fortunate our little girl had survived at all. Every day that passed, her chances improved.

The staff of the special care unit were like gods to us in those first hours and days. We felt helpless and trusted in them completely to care for our Megan. We were encouraged to touch her immediately. We held her feet with one hand and the top of her head with the other. We were told all about kangaroo care and couldn't wait to hold her.

On the third day I was released from the hospital. It was horribly painful to leave without her that night. I felt so empty. I wanted to live at the hospital until she was able to come home, too. I had been away from home for only a few days, yet my entire world had changed. I recall driving up to the house and feeling so strange, as if I didn't belong there. It did become easier as we developed a daily routine, but every night I wished I could be with her. The thought of her lying there alone was heartbreaking. I also went through a period of a week or two in which I had very intense feelings that

Megan was mine alone. I wanted her completely to myself. David and I joke that it is a good thing those feelings began *after* I had filled out the birth certificate; otherwise, the father's name probably would have been left blank!

Megan's fourth day was a very special one. Her second head ultrasound came back clear—no brain bleeds found so far. Her cultures came back negative—no infections detected—and she was taken off antibiotics. That day Megan was also taken off dopamine, which had been used to stabilize her blood pressure. She received her first lipids intravenously. The most wonderful thing that happened, however, was being asked by the nurse when we arrived that morning whether I wanted to kangaroo with my daughter. I hadn't thought I'd be able to hold her for a couple of weeks! She was so fragile, so small. I recall her tiny hand lying on my chest. I cannot describe the feeling the first time I held her against my skin, how amazing it was. I never wanted it to end. It was the first time I really felt like a mother. David, too, was able to kangaroo her that afternoon. From that day on we each looked forward to kangarooing with our little girl every day. We talked to her and sang to her. We rubbed the tape on her cheek that held her tubes in place. She really enjoyed that. (We always imagined that the tape made her skin very itchy.) I recall sometimes feeling very impatient when the nurse was not able to prepare Megan to be removed from her isolette immediately. Every minute that went by was lost kangarooing time. I think that kangarooing was just as important for David as it was for me, although he often let me have extra kangaroo turns. I had been able to express breast milk for Megan, whereas kangaroo care was something very special that David could do for Megan.

Finally, on day five, Megan was breathing on her own. She had suffered from respiratory distress syndrome, though she was on a ventilator for only one day. She needed only two doses of Surfactant for her lungs, received theophylline for thirty-seven days, and respiratory therapy (chest vibes) for her lungs, which she did not like at all. Megan had jaundice and was under bilirubin lights for fifteen days. She was also anemic. She had an umbilical artery catheter for drawing blood gases because her tiny peripheral veins were collapsing from the intravenous tubes. The neonatologist designated a potential undamaged site on Megan's arm to remain free of IVs in case she required a more permanent and more risky cut-down line, which, fortunately, she never needed. Her final IV location was in her scalp. Thankfully, we were warned before we saw her with the IV in her head, and nursery staff assured us that this IV site was harder for parents than for the babies. By day ten Megan was no longer receiving anything intravenously. The only things attached to her were her monitors and a nasogastric tube.

I was very anxious around the monitors in the Special Care Nursery. The nurses noted that sometimes I spent more time staring at the monitors than looking at my baby. For a time I lived in terror of those things and the apnea and bradycardia episodes that they announced. When the alarms went off, the nurses would assess the situation and usually determine that everything was fine. Then they would tell me to look at my baby, watch her breathe, and look at the color of her skin. They taught me to interpret the monitors in conjunction with one another in order to determine if there was really a problem. By the time Megan was released, I was much calmer about the alarms. After we brought her home, their advice to "look at my baby" was very useful. In the early weeks I had frequent fears, especially at night, that she had stopped breathing. I was able to look at her and feel assured.

During her stay in the Special Care Nursery we became obsessed with Megan's weight. After six days her weight had declined to 977 grams (2 pounds 2.5 ounces)—a decline of almost 15 percent of her birth weight. She was weighed each night during the overnight shift. I eagerly phoned the nursery each night to ask about her weight. On the fifteenth day Megan surpassed her birth weight! From then on it was an almost constant climb. At first even a single gram was cause for celebration. As time went on, an increase of less than 20 grams was a disappointment. I made a graph of her weight gain that I updated each morning. David created a Web site where he posted photos of Megan and updated her weight each day. Our family and friends were able to check on her from the Web site.

When Megan first arrived in the Special Care Nursery, she was the smallest, gestationally youngest, and highest-need baby there. About two weeks later, a twenty-five-week higher-need baby boy arrived in the nursery. That day, I am ashamed to say, I felt disappointment that Megan was no longer the worst case in the nursery. I did not want her level of care to decrease for any reason. That little boy had a tougher time than Megan. I watched his parents suffer like no other parents in the nursery at the time. When their son hit a tough spot, they sometimes asked us if Megan had experienced the same problem, but she usually hadn't. I wished I could help them somehow because I knew they were even more frightened than we were. That little boy overcame many challenges. The last time I heard, he was doing great. I think about him often.

At some point the question changed from "Will my baby survive?" to "Will my baby be okay?" Somewhere in there the pedestal on which I had placed the special care staff became somewhat shaky. They were real people. I trusted many of the nurses without question. I felt less confident in a few others for one reason or another. Most of the nurses were open to our concerns or requests, and although we were encouraged to take an active role in Megan's care, as time went on it was very difficult to leave our daughter in the care of others when, ultimately, she was our responsibility.

There were a few things about the nursery in general that we wish had been different. It was sometimes unnecessarily loud and bright. The charge nurses, through no fault of their own, sometimes spent as much time dealing with staffing issues as attending to the babies. Our experience, however, was very positive. We learned so much about caring for Megan from the skilled and compassionate nurses. In fact, the Special Care Nursery became our world. We sometimes wondered what we would do with ourselves at home alone, without the expertise, support, and friendship of the hospital staff. We would miss so many people, from the receptionist at the maternity ward desk to the wonderful lactation consultants who worked with us long after Megan's discharge, to the caring young woman who cleaned the hospital rooms. We could barely remember what life was like before. Also, although I understand that many babies come through the Special Care Nursery, I didn't want them to forget Megan. The Special Care Nursery was indeed a special place. I still think about our friends there every day. We have visited the nursery several times since Megan's discharge seven months ago, and, interestingly, I don't feel that we belong there anymore. I guess that is the way it should be.

I began expressing breast milk with an electric pump a few hours after Megan's birth. I had planned to nurse, and the hospital staff stressed how vital breast milk is for premature infants. I found pumping awkward and painful at first. For the first day or two I didn't even collect enough to pour into a container. By the second night I collected 3 centimeters into a container and proudly brought it to the nursery. I was so happy. I felt that I could finally do something for my baby. The nursery staff was so gracious about my modest deposit. They placed it in the freezer to save for when Megan would be able to eat through a nasogastric tube. They acted about as excited as I was. Our first attempt at nuzzling at the breast during kangaroo care took place on the tenth day. It was promising. Megan seemed to have the idea, and I gained some confidence. In a later attempt on the twenty-second day, Megan actually got some milk and didn't know what to do with it. She choked and had a bradycardia.

On day thirty-two, Megan's first oral feeding was planned, despite the objection of one of the lead nurses who felt it was too soon. The bottle was filled with 30 cc's of breast milk. The neonatologist warned that it was just an experiment and not to expect much. Well, our little baby outdid herself! She took 15 cc's. We were elated. The next day our nursing effort began in earnest. A few sessions went well, but overall she showed little ability to nurse. The bottle feeding wasn't going well, either. Megan had met and overcome so many challenges. We never expected oral feeding to be such an issue. The NG tube was the primary method of feeding her until three days prior to her discharge from the hospital.

Breast-feeding was my primary focus during the latter part of Megan's time in special care. I really wanted to nurse full-time. I was concerned about the bond between my daughter and me after so much time apart. I also wanted to provide her with the best possible nutrition since she had been cheated out of so much time in the womb. For several weeks I got up at 3 A.M. to go to the hospital to nurse. I worked from 6:30 A.M. to 12:30 P.M. and returned to the hospital for her afternoon feeding. At the very end, the hospital kindly allowed me to spend the night in a hospital room so that I could nurse her more often. I was pumping every two to three hours around the clock. I was absolutely exhausted, and I wanted my relationship with the breast pump to end. I kept telling myself that I only needed to hold out until she came home, then she would nurse and it would be so much easier. Nine months later, I am still pumping. Megan was only able to nurse on a limited basis when she came home. We rented a digital scale and measured exactly how much she nursed each session. The most she ever took at one feeding was 80 cc's. Feedings were such an ordeal. We would nurse, I would follow up with a bottle of previously expressed milk, and then I would pump. She was eating about every two hours, so it was almost a continuous process. Soon I gave up even trying to nurse her during the night. Now I wish I had tried harder.

By Megan's due date, feeding by breast or bottle became a serious struggle. She seemed very hungry but refused the bottle. She would thrash around and scream. Her first pediatrician suggested that Megan must not like breast milk and instructed us, despite my objections, to give her formula and force her to eat. Regrettably, we actually tried that for a couple of days. She continued to reject the bottle and ate very little. We promptly found a new pediatrician who immediately identified a feeding problem. It has been suggested that her feeding difficulties were the result of oral feeding too early; maybe that nurse was right after all!

Megan spent sixty-three days in the Special Care Nursery. There were many special days as she reached important milestones that all preemies go through: breathing on her own, surpassing her birth weight, moving from a radiant warmer to an isolette and from an isolette to an open bassinet, and her first feeding by mouth. Another special day was Halloween. When I arrived at the nursery that afternoon, I was surprised to find my tiny baby girl dressed up in the cutest little clown costume, matching hat and all! David had shopped all over looking for a costume for her. He even considered having one custom made. He finally found just what he was looking for in a doll shop. I had had no idea what he was up to. He even asked a nurse to videotape me as I walked in. Even better, the nurses were so excited by Megan's costume that they made impromptu costumes for all the other babies, too. What a great day! Another special day was Megan's two-month birthday. It was the day before her release. We brought lunch and a cake to celebrate with the nursery staff and the other parents—a combination birthday party and farewell. When we went into the nursery that morning, there was a birthday sign posted above Megan's bed that was signed by the nurses and other staff. It was such a happy day!

While Megan was in the Special Care Nursery, I thought that everything would be easier as soon as we could bring her home. We would not need to shuttle back and forth from work to hospital to home. We would not worry about her being alone because we would be with her. We would get more sleep. I was very wrong. About three weeks after Megan came home, just around her due date, she became a very high need baby. She became easily "disorganized" and needed David or me to soothe her. We were not prepared for the change. We literally became human mattresses as we took turns kangarooing to comfort her at night. During the day she wanted to be held all the time, but simply holding her wasn't enough. I had to walk or dance and sing much of the day. This was all in between the every-two-hour feeding cycle. In addition, I still needed to pump every two or three hours in order to maintain my milk supply. This was difficult because Megan did not want to be put down *ever*. When David came home from work, he took over. We were completely run down.

Megan is still a high-need baby but, over time, the situation has significantly improved. She now wakes only once during the night to eat. We have learned what helps: baths, massage, a front-carrying or hip baby carrier, any kind of movement, recorded music, and singing special songs. As her motor skills have progressed, she has become somewhat less dependent on us to soothe her.

We have been very fortunate. Megan did not suffer from many of the more serious problems that preemies are prone to. She had no brain bleeds, no infections, needed little supplemental oxygen, underwent no surgical procedures, and required no blood transfusions. She is now nine months old and is a bright, beautiful, and very happy baby. She has passed initial hearing and vision screenings. She appears to have no cognitive problems. Her gross motor skills are somewhat delayed, however, even for her corrected age. She is under the expert care of a supportive pediatrician and highly talented therapists, and is fully expected to catch up. We are forever grateful for the invaluable support and kindness we have received from so many people and are especially indebted to the wonderful people from Special

Care and from Easter Seals who cared not only for Megan but for her parents as well.

Megan's Prayer

BY GLORIA L. ETES

Dear Lord,
Listen to my little prayer
For the wonderful folks in "Special Care."
As every sparrow's fall you see,
Watch over them as they did me.
For they kept me clean and fed,
Rubbed my chest and soothed my head,
Charted every cough and sneeze,
Monitored my A's and B's.
Hope in Mom and Dad maintained.
Thrilled with every gram I gained.
My nursery pals were all aware
Of their tender, ever-present care.
To help me grow up to repay
And bring their love to others someday.
Amen

Written for Megan Elizabeth Redheffer-Fickert
Born September 16, 1997, 2 pounds 8 ounces

FEELINGS OF A PREEMIE PARENT

by Terry Tremethick

I personally think our emotions are the most complex part of us. We react to everything around us with certain feelings—sometimes ones we are unaware of. Parents of premature babies react like anyone else. The feelings we experience are normal but often not understood by others around us. Let's face it: Everyone knows someone who has had a premature baby, but not as many actually have had one themselves.

I will share with you what my wife, Karla, and I felt and how we dealt—or failed to deal—with the many emotions we experienced and still are experiencing. Each of us is an individual, but it would be foolish to assume no one else has felt what I have felt or gone through what I have. In the final analysis, we are very alike in the way we feel.

Initial Shock

The first emotion I felt was shock—utter disbelief—at seeing this tiny out-of-proportion baby that did not resemble a newborn. We had been through the mill for almost five weeks prior to the birth and were already in a drained emotional state.

What should we feel? We were in new territory. How can you know how you will react under pressure if you have not experienced it? A friend who spent some time in the U.S. Army told me only 10 percent of soldiers actually fire back effectively during battle. Why? Because of pressure they hadn't had to cope with previously. I suppose they are shocked. People congratulated us, sent us flowers, and patted me on the back, and asked me how it was to be a father. We did not want any of these things because we were in shock. Our baby was very sick, and that was all that occupied our thoughts.

Disappointment and Grief

We felt disappointed that we had been robbed of a normal pregnancy. You know the story: Both of you are told you are going to have a baby, and you are given a due date. When the baby suddenly comes really early, you feel that disappointment. You see other mothers with their children happy and playing, and your thoughts go to your little one in intensive care. Karla said she often felt "ripped off" because she had not experienced all the wonders of pregnancy she had expected. It is all about expecting certain things and their not happening at all or the way you think they should be.

A child should not come into the world three months early. The child should still be in its mother's womb, growing and being nurtured in a beautiful way that only a mother can give it. The womb is awesome, and no amount of advanced equipment can come anywhere near it! When you see your baby struggling because he or she is not meant to be here yet, the pang of hurt inside you is enormous. I can only guess how much worse it must be for a mother.

Anger

Here is that emotion that is thrown around so much these days. Once you get over the initial shock and then disappointment, the next thing that will probably knock on your heart's door will be anger. This was a very difficult one for me. You find yourself lashing out at people and situations for no reason at all. We both were angry about what was happening. You feel so helpless that the only response you can find is anger—anger at the world, anger at others who seem less deserving, and anger at yourself because you can do nothing to change what has occurred. However, anger is dangerous if left unchecked. We had to talk constantly to each other about what we were feeling. That was the key for us, not to let it burn inside and build up. We are all human, and I know I had so much anger that it was turning to bitterness. I had to let it go. Face it first, and then let it go. Easier said than done.

Not Alone

What made it easier? We felt we were not alone. We knew God was somehow looking after us, and this brought amazing peace. Why had He let it happen? I threw this question at God many times. I do not understand why, only that I had two choices: bitterness or letting it go. I don't intend to get all religious here. Many people who cared supported us—and still do—not in a passing way but in a real way. Sometimes all you need is someone to listen or just be a friend without actually saying anything. We found talking about anything else helped because the constant questions about the trauma seemed to make it look bigger and more painful.

What Then?

There is nothing Karla and I could do about our feelings. Denial only made it worse. What would we say to you now if you were going through this experience? Don't get bitter and don't isolate yourself. Find real friends to ease the burden. Couples should talk to each other about it. All very simple. I am not a therapist. I only share with you our experience. We were not the first, and we will not be the last. There is probably someone much worse off.

HER GRANDFATHER ANGEL WAS WATCHING: SENIA'S STORY

by Kimberly A. Powell

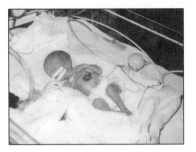

Senia, eight hours old.

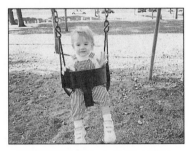

Senia, seventeen months old.

One of the first cards we received after our daughter was born was a sympathy card that read:

> *Warm thoughts are with you . . .*
> *There is so little*
> *one can say,*
> *so little one can do,*
> *But may it comfort*
> *you to know*
> *that thoughts go out*
> *to you.*

No, our daughter did not die at birth. Our daughter was premature—
twelve weeks premature. Senia entered our lives at a tiny 1 pound 15
ounces on March 3, 1997. Although not as we had planned her birth,
this was a joyous though shocking time of our lives.

My earliest memories include the lack of any desire to have children. On April 21, 1996, my desires changed due to a life-altering
event: death. On April 21 my father-in-law, Glenn Sikkink, died
suddenly of a heart attack in the middle of the night. As the family
gathered in the emergency room of the hospital, I began to change.
The outpouring of love and support rooted in this close family
planted a seed in me, a seed of desire to have a child and expand our
family. The ability of a tragic event to spawn life out of death is both
miraculous and curious.

We found out in September 1996 that we were pregnant. Our excitement was fueled by the fact that this was a perfectly timed pregnancy. The baby was due on May 22, immediately following the end
of the semester at the college at which I taught. Knowing the timing
was perfect, we were free to spend the next months anticipating the
birth of our baby. I loved being pregnant! Going through each day
knowing I had a tiny life growing inside me was a joy. I would imagine how my baby looked, her personality, her likes and dislikes. All
of this was possible because I was having the perfect pregnancy—
perfect until February 27, 1997.

I was entering the third trimester of my pregnancy and feeling
great through aerobics class on Monday and a circuit training work-
out on Tuesday. On Wednesday I planned to teach my three classes,
go to aerobics, and then to my monthly prenatal exam. This was
when the gestational diabetes test would be done. Diabetes runs in
my family, so although I felt great, I was a bit nervous about the results of this test. My husband and I entered the office full of nervous
excitement. This excitement quickly waned as the nurse took my
blood pressure, 140/90. I never had high blood pressure, so this reading was high enough for worry. When my urine test showed protein,

the doctor drew some blood for tests and I was sent home on bed rest immediately. My doctor said it was possible I had developed preeclampsia, but she wanted to see me in two days to check my blood pressure again; perhaps the rise was due to my nervousness over the gestational diabetes test. As I drove home in tears, asking "Why me?" I developed the sinking feeling that there was a serious problem with my pregnancy, one that a day of bed rest would not cure.

The dreaded phone call came the next day. I did not have gestational diabetes and did not need to return to the doctor for a blood pressure check on Friday. I was to be admitted to the hospital as soon as possible for fetal monitoring and a twenty-four-hour urine count. As my husband and I sat in the hospital watching the fetal monitor, we were in a state of disbelief. Surely I would be sent home that evening. Reality began to set in when my doctor told us the baby was doing fine but she was worried about my life. I spent the next two nights in our small-town hospital listening to three women go through full-term labor and delivery, amid my hourly blood pressure checks and fetal monitoring. As I heard the first cries of mother and child, my eyes filled with tears of fear and sadness. Why could my pregnancy not go to term? I had eaten right, exercised, and maintained my good health, so why me?

The news got progressively worse as I was transferred to a larger hospital seventy-five minutes away from home. This facility was equipped with preeclampsia specialists and an excellent NICU. While being in a better facility was reassuring, I was being moved away from my husband and friends for a projected three to four weeks on bed rest. The loneliness quickly set in. No longer was I in familiar surroundings; I was in a sterile environment trying to postpone the birth of my baby. How strange it seemed to be trying to prolong meeting the child I had bonded with and looked forward to helping into this world. As I lay on my left side in bed over the next two days, I read much on labor and delivery, as my Lamaze class was not planned to start for another two weeks. The staff tried to keep my spirits up with frequent visits, videos, books, and a tour of the NICU that would serve as my baby's first home. Seeing the 4-pound babies living in the NICU alleviated my fears. These were such cute little people with only a couple of wires attached to monitor their breathing and heart rate. Unfortunately for me, these babies did not even slightly resemble my tiny being who was born the next day.

On Monday I was scheduled for an ultrasound at 8:30 A.M. to determine how much oxygen my baby was getting. The angels were watching, for the technicians were behind schedule. I waited in my hospital room until they came for me at 2:30 P.M.—the last time I would be in my room as a pregnant woman. As I was being wheeled to the ultrasound room, I began feeling light-headed but knew this was a symptom of high blood pressure, so I did not worry. Once we reached the ultrasound room, I felt a sudden pain in my upper abdomen like nothing I had experienced before. The technician diagnosed the pain as indigestion, but I knew I could not possibly have eaten anything to cause indigestion this severe. I began throwing up, sweating profusely, and complaining of an intense headache. The technician called in the doctor who, knowing my preeclampsia had progressed to a severe stage, pronounced that my pregnancy had to be over in two hours if the baby and I were to live. I had HELLP syndrome (hemolysis, elevated liver enzymes, and low blood platelets). Suddenly my perfect pregnancy and joys of having a child turned to pain, fear, and chaos.

The next few hours were so full of activity that it took weeks for me to piece the events together. In the midst of all my pain, worries about my baby, and wishing my husband had been notified in time to be by my side, the reality that I was about to be a mother never sunk in. The third trimester was to be the time for me and my husband to prepare ourselves mentally and the house physically for our new addition. Two hours were just not sufficient. The last hours of my pregnancy were spent with a blood pressure of 220/180, severe headaches leading to seizure, an expanding liver causing the severe abdominal pain, a catheter, an IV, and medication that sent a fire through my body to stop seizures; it was administered every minute through a shunt in my hand. In the midst of this chaos I remember thinking how "normal" this day was for the people working around me. While my life and the life of my child were in danger, I remember the nurses talking about who would stay late and what they had planned for their evenings, but mostly I remember being asked in the middle of the ordeal to sign a consent form—as if I was coherent enough to make such a decision. In the face of death, life went on.

Once the anesthesia took effect, in preparation for my child being taken from me by cesarean section, my becoming a parent still was not a reality. My only thoughts were of the desire to be out of pain and of the location of my husband. The joy of childbirth was taken from me: no labor, no anticipation, no being one of the first to see my child, no cradling my baby in my arms once she had been taken from her warm womb home.

After thirty-six hours on magnesium sulfate, unable to move a muscle in my body, my first meeting with my baby was to take place. My husband had arrived fifteen minutes after the birth and was shocked to learn he was a father and the circumstances of the birth. He spent the hours after our daughter's birth shuttling between the NICU and my recovery room. Although he brought me pictures of our baby, I was not prepared for the tiny creature I was to meet. Once my body had calmed down, I was wheeled into the NICU on my hospital bed to meet my daughter. After being assured that I was still seeing double from the magnesium and did not have twins, I focused on a baby smaller than any I had ever seen: Her head was the size of a baseball; my husband's wedding ring fit around her biceps; her fingers and toes were long and skinny like a bird's claws; and her ribs were protected by nothing more than purple skin clinging to her bones. Once internalizing her size, I could focus on how perfect she was. Though tiny, she was a complete, perfect little girl. How could a baby so small be so perfect? How could a baby so perfect but small live? As my baby lay on her bed warmer, connected to a respirator, monitor, and IV, she wrapped her tiny fingers around the tip of my finger, and I felt she knew me.

We named our baby Senia Glenn after her great-great aunt and her late grandfather, the reason for her being. As I recovered and walked the hall from my room to the NICU several times a day, I still could not tell well-wishers who Senia looked like or how it felt to hold her. I could not because I did not know. While parents of full-term babies quickly decide who the baby looks like, parents of preemies cannot. My baby was a tiny being composed of skin and bones, with the tape that held the respirator in her mouth covering her features. I did not know whose nose she had, whose mouth she had, or that she had any features resembling anyone. They were not noticeable under the tape, beneath the wires, in the isolette, under the bilirubin lights. Not having held her, I not only did not know how to describe her but I had not bonded with her. I was so mentally unprepared and so ill that I had not yet realized I was a mom and Senia was my daughter. I knew I loved my baby more than anything in the world and wanted her to live, but I did not feel connected to her. Holding her instantaneously connected us.

Three days after her birth, the nurses asked if I wanted to hold my daughter. Yes, I wanted to hold her, but I was afraid. How does one hold a 1-pound-12-ounce baby? I could not just pick her up and cradle her. She was so fragile and breakable that I feared harming her. The nurses assured me that kangaroo holding was beneficial to both Senia and me, so I lay back perfectly still in a recliner while three nurses organized the wires and the respirator to work Senia out of her isolette and onto the bare skin of my chest. As she settled onto me, skin to skin, and grabbed my finger, I could not control the tears. My daughter did not hate me for not being able to keep her in her cozy womb home. She loved and knew me. From that moment on, Senia and I were bonded for life.

Over the next weeks of traveling the seventy-five minutes to the hospital almost daily, we slowly began to realize we were parents and that our daughter was going to come home one day. Life in a NICU is a roller coaster. One day your baby is doing well, the next she has taken a turn for the worse. One Saturday, three weeks after Senia's birth, the phone rang, and it was the NICU. My heart sank as they asked for permission to have a surgeon insert a lifeline because Senia's previous two IVs had become infected. Knowing the surgeon was the same one who performed her late grandfather's heart surgery twelve years before, we felt her grandfather angel was watching. I gave my permission, and I was warned that she was very tired and I should not expect much from my visit. When I arrived at the hospital later that afternoon, I found my daughter limp and lifeless. The infection had taken its toll, resulting in her forgetting to breathe approximately every twenty minutes. The nurse encouraged me to hold Senia briefly, hoping that would help comfort her. Senia stopped breathing six times during the twenty minutes that I held her. Each time that the bag ventilator was used to make Senia breathe, my heart fell. I left the hospital knowing my daughter's life was out of my hands, and I feared I might lose her. This was the first time since her birth that I allowed myself to cry out of the fear of losing the daughter I wanted and loved so much. Fortunately, the next day the antibiotics and new lifeline worked. That day Senia opened her eyes and gave us her first smile. The projection was smooth sailing. We had only to wait for Senia to be able to eat enough by mouth to gain weight, and to be able to take in enough oxygen to avoid desaturations.

As I sat in the NICU with Senia I saw many babies come and go. Senia went from being the only baby in the NICU to one of thirteen, and finally one of three. Would it ever be our turn to go home? I began to think I would never get to hold my baby like a full-term baby, much less be able to walk anywhere with her without an oxygen machine and monitor. It became painful to be around other new mothers and babies. I wanted my baby home. Senia had been in the

NICU for weeks. The biggest hurdle for Senia now was her breathing. Though I had been given steroid shots before her birth to speed up their development and she had been given two doses of Surfactant, her lungs were still not mature enough to take in the oxygen her body needed. She was having frequent desaturations on 30 percent oxygen. The doctors decided to give Senia a seven-day dose of the steroid Decadron to speed up her lung development. They felt the risks of high blood sugar and mood changes were outweighed by the benefits of getting Senia off the oxygen, which would decrease her risks of eye problems.

After three days the Decadron appeared to be working; Senia began having fewer desaturations—though she had some moody days! Senia also began taking more milk by mouth, which decreased the amount of nutrients she needed through her lifeline. Actually, Senia was drinking more breast milk than I was producing. Since I had been so sick, my milk did not come in for three weeks, and when it did, I was excited if I produced 1 ounce. This 1 ounce per pumping was sufficient to feed Senia for the first five weeks of her life, for she started on only half a cc an hour of one-quarter-strength breast milk. I can laugh now when I think back to my little bag of breast milk in the NICU freezer surrounded by gallons of milk the other mothers were producing. Although Senia was having fewer desaturations and was eating more, losing her was still a possibility. Gradually, our hopes began to outweigh our fears, and we began to let ourselves plan for her homecoming. We bought furniture and diapers, decorated Senia's room, and friends threw a baby shower. We were now doing what we had planned to do in the third trimester.

April 11 was liberation day for Senia in many ways. Her lifeline came out, she was taking all food by mouth, and she finally moved from the incubator to a crib. Three days later she was to come off oxygen. During the last ten days of Senia's hospital stay, I stayed with her, which allowed me to become comfortable caring for her.

Until this time I was afraid to move her by myself, to change her diaper alone, or to feed her without supervision. Actually staying with Senia made me feel for the first time that I was really a mother. For the first time I was giving my baby all her feedings, changing all her diapers, comforting her when she cried, rocking her to sleep, and giving her a mother's tender loving care. Until now I had been a visitor; now I was a mother. When the day finally came to take Senia home, I was ready.

On April 21, one year to the day of her grandfather Glenn's death, Senia came home. At 4 pounds 1 ounce, the apnea and bradycardia monitor Senia came home on was heavier than she was. For the next two and a half months Senia had frequent apneas and bradycardias, which scared us greatly; however, she worked her way off the monitor as she passed her due date. Though we could not have visitors or take Senia out to show her off until a month past her due date for fear of infection, we were very proud parents. Despite leaping out of bed at night to the sound of the monitor, checking Senia's breathing several times an hour, worrying about infection, and missing the security of the NICU nurses, we were overjoyed to have our baby home. No more long rides to the hospital, no more machine sounds, no more waking up at night wishing our baby was in her room. Senia was home.

Now that Senia is a healthy and growing two-year-old, I look back on her preemie experience as a special time of watching my daughter develop. Though I would not have chosen to have a child early, I had the unique opportunity to watch my child develop much as she would have in the womb. Premature children are special, determined little miracles—miracles aided by many very special NICU nurses and doctors. My little miracle will always know she lived and thrived because of the help of these angels and her special grandfather angel.

OUR LIVES ARE CHANGED FOREVER: SARAH'S LESSONS

by Deborah Broad-Erickson

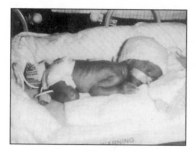

Sarah, one day old.

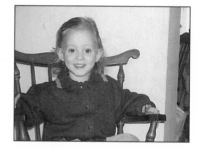

Sarah, thirty-three months old.

Being pregnant with Sarah was a highlight in my life. Although at the beginning I would have sworn that "she" was a "he," I was thrilled to know that there was a little baby growing inside me. After losing our first baby at thirteen weeks, my husband, Rijon, and I knew about loss—now we wanted to know about parenthood. My pregnancy was regarded as high risk due to the first miscarriage and the development of a blood disorder called autoimmune thrombocy-topenia purpura, or ATP. (Simply put, there was an antibody that was slowly killing off the platelets that clotted blood in my body.) All of this made for a pregnancy full of questions and concern.

Our monthly visits with Sarah via ultrasound were very exciting. To watch her heart beat and see her growing calmed me more than any words a doctor could speak. My platelet disorder was monitored with monthly blood tests. I looked forward to routine visits twice a month to my OB-GYN and once to a perinatologist, when I would hear Sarah's heart beating through the Doppler. Things were going well for a high-risk pregnancy until the end of month six. An ultrasound showed Sarah's growth had slowed, and she was small for her gestational age. Bed rest was ordered, as were betamethasone steroid shots to help mature Sarah's lungs. The plan was, as the doctor had said, "to keep this baby in until thirty-five weeks." "Her name is Sarah" was my reply. HELLP syndrome was not even in my vocabulary at that time; now I know it intimately. HELLP, which stands for hemolysis (breakdown of red blood cells), elevated liver enzymes, and low platelets, is a variant of severe preeclampsia that I was never made aware of. I was just getting over the shock of learning about intrauterine growth restriction (IUGR) and that my body, no matter how well I ate, was not nourishing our baby due to placental breakdown. I was blindsided by this new syndrome.

I was introduced to HELLP at 1 A.M. on June 11 when I awoke with pain in what is called the upper right quadrant, just below the rib cage. By 3 A.M. I was in so much pain that I was startled by my own voice moaning as I lay in the darkness. We were staying at my parents' home because my husband was leaving on a business trip that morning and I had just begun bed rest. Rijon was fast asleep and I did not want to wake him, but by 5 A.M. I could not keep from vomiting and was hoping he would hear me. I was scared by what was happening. Instead my mother came and brought me to my old bedroom where she tucked me into bed. She did not want to wake the others, including my younger sister and her husband who were expecting their first baby, now nearly one week overdue.

Over the course of the next day I was in and out of consciousness, vomiting and in such pain that before my mother left for work, I grabbed hold of her arm and thanked her for taking care of me. She nodded and smiled but then asked me why I was saying that now. "I am dying, Mom," I said. "Really, I feel that I am going to die today." She had no idea that I was dangerously close to the truth. By 4:30 P.M. my father, who had come home so my mother could work, persuaded me to phone the obstetrician on call. I had learned over the months of pregnancy that certain doctors in the practice did not take my concerns seriously, and although my mother had begged me all morning to call the doctor, it was best to try to handle situations alone rather than be made to feel by the OB-GYN that I was a hypochondriac. I described the situation to the doctor, saying I was very weak and dehydrated, and he told me to take some antacid—his remedy for everything. I told him that I had tried this and that it had not worked. Begrudgingly, he told me to head to the hospital where he would have a resident take a look at me.

When I arrived at the hospital, the resident smirked and asked if I had missed them. I had been seen just two days prior for back, chest, and abdominal pain, which may have been the first signs of my body rebelling against the baby. My feeling of vindication came as this same resident watched me vomit uncontrollably. She knew I was not "faking." It was not a physician who saved me, however; it was my father who noted that I looked jaundiced or "yellow." This observation set the doctors in motion, and tests were done to check my liver enzymes. Sure enough, every count was elevated except for my platelets, which were dropping. During the next five hours I was poked and prodded, was in and out of consciousness, but never received anything to dull my abdominal pain because this would have made it harder for the doctors to know if my condition was worsening. My mother arrived at the hospital at 10 P.M., and I looked into her eyes as I listened to my obstetrician tell me that I had preeclampsia and that I would be kept in the hospital for four weeks until the baby could be delivered.

Through the night I saw many faces hovering over me as I lay in bed in the high-risk ward: my perinatologist, other doctors, and nurses. The same fetal monitors that were telling me Sarah was fine were pressing on my expanding liver and causing greater pain, and I thrashed about trying to escape their pressure. At 3 A.M. I told the nurse that I could not take anymore, and although I did not know it then, she already knew I was going downhill fast. I was whisked away to labor and delivery. My family was called, and they paged my husband, who was hundreds of miles away.

I was prepped for an emergency cesarean section by a very kind nurse. She continued to tell me that the baby looked good (from the monitors), and I told her "the baby" was named Sarah. From then on that nurse called my baby by her name. My family gathered around my bed—some crying, others rubbing the sleep from their eyes, all assuring me I was going to be all right. The lab results showed something different. My liver enzymes skyrocketed, and the organ itself was estimated at three times its normal size. Also, a bleeding test was administered, and in fifteen minutes my blood never clotted, not even once. The obstetrician came into the room. My coworkers had been right: Of all the doctors in the practice, the one you dislike the most will be the one to deliver your baby. There he stood in front of me, but not as cocky-looking now that his coat and tie were replaced by scrubs. He looked young, which he was, and he looked sorry. Perhaps he was—for not believing what I had known—that I was a lot sicker than he thought. He apologized for what he was about to tell me. They could not wait for Rijon to arrive. The baby had to come out immediately, and the procedure would be a classic c-section with no hope of ever delivering vaginally in the future. Finally, I would not be awake for Sarah's birth because an epidural could cause me to bleed to death. Instead, I would be under general anesthesia and transfused with platelets to help me clot during the surgery. I nodded to him and then, after a short goodbye to my family, was wheeled into the surgical room. I was almost frantic as fear overtook me. My pain, however, was gone. I no longer felt the acute ache in my liver that had been there for over twenty-four hours. The anesthesiologist placed a mask over my face for the gas they would use, and my throat tightened. My arms had been placed straight out from my body on boards, and I was very uncomfortable. I was told to take deep breaths of the anesthetic gas and relax.

It was 5:53 A.M. when Sarah was born. She weighed 1 pound 12 ounces and measured 12⅝ inches long. I felt as if I had been hit by a truck when I slowly opened my eyes. My family was with me as I lay in recovery, and finally at 9 A.M. Rijon arrived. Sarah was in the NICU, and all I had were two pictures of her. I could not fully comprehend that she had been born, and instead of demanding to see her, I slept. Finally, that evening, Rijon brought in a hospital VCR and showed me a videotape of little Sarah; he had filmed her as she lay in her isolette. Still it all seemed unreal. The next day brought more tests for me and for Sarah. A decision needed to be made about a blood vessel outside Sarah's heart that had not closed, called a PDA, and we had to consent to medical treatment that would be tried before possible surgery. As I lay in intensive care recovery, I barely knew what to say about this, my first decision as a parent. Drowsily, I looked up at Rijon and told him to do whatever he felt was best.

That evening I was to visit Sarah for the first time. I was carefully loaded into a wheelchair and taken down corridor after corridor. Rijon maneuvered down the halls as if he knew them like the back of his hand—and he did; he had been to the NICU many times in the past two days. Rijon picked up the phone outside the NICU. I listened as he said, "Rijon and Debbie Erickson to see our daughter, Sarah." The words seemed to hit me as he spoke them: We have a daughter. She is here, she is here.

Rijon showed me how to "scrub in," and I was nearly soaked as I tried to wash from my wheelchair. I read the words on the door we were about to enter: Neonatal Intensive Care Unit. I said to myself, "My life is about to change forever." Once inside, I slowly passed many isolettes. I thought each one was where we were stopping, and

I would ask, "Is this her?" Finally we did stop, and I looked around. Monitors beeping, nurses everywhere, wires, tubes, and there was Sarah. I wanted to cry, I wanted to smile, to feel something, but I was numb, I was in shock. It was only when I read her name on the little pink card on her isolette and looked at her tiny fingers that I realized this was my daughter and she was really here. Rijon showed me the hand holes in the side of the isolette, and I reached inside. Softly, gently, I began to stroke Sarah's little leg. A hand firmly grasped my arm, and I stopped and looked up. "Don't touch her like that," said the nurse by my side. "Her central nervous system is underdeveloped and cannot tolerate being touched lightly. Instead, cup your hands and place one hand around her head and one around her bottom." Tears sprang to my eyes, and my mind raced: How dare this nurse tell me how to touch! I was not stupid. I had held many babies. I knew how to touch babies! But I did not know how to touch, feed, turn, or cuddle a premature baby. All of this I learned over the next ten weeks.

I learned many other things as well. As a person who feels the need for control in her life, I realized that I had none in the NICU. When Sarah contracted a staph infection at two weeks old, called methacillin resistant staph aureus (MRSA), and another at six weeks, called necrotizing enterocolitis (NEC), I asked my rabbi what to do—tell Sarah to stop fighting or encourage her to keep going. He told me, "Sarah will do what she has to do no matter what you tell her. Your job is to tell her you love her and to be there for her. She will do what she needs to do." As a young woman I had to learn about accepting that not all dreams come true. I had dreamt of the perfect delivery with my husband by my side, bonding after Sarah's birth and nursing her. I had to come to terms with the way everything unfolded and take pride in the fact that I did breast-feed Sarah, if only by way of a mechanical pump and a nurse with a gavage tube. I learned that not everyone can empathize with me and understand the pain I felt. A surgeon who was observing Sarah after she was transferred to a children's hospital because of NEC spoke to me very harshly. I asked him how he could be so blunt and so mean. He told me that he was just doing his job and that if he looked at every baby he operated on as someone's child, he would be too emotionally involved to operate on them. "What do you want, Mrs. Erickson? For me to cry with you or to save your daughter's life?"

Another lesson came from my sister, Beth, who gave birth to a healthy 8-pound-14-ounce son named Joshua. During this very hard time when, because of stress and other factors, my body stopped producing milk for Sarah, my sister generously donated some of her own breast milk for my daughter to use before she was placed on formula. Even though this time was very difficult for everyone, our family never abandoned us.

Sarah will be two years old soon. She is still underweight but doing very well, and we know that we are extremely lucky. HELLP syndrome and Sarah's prematurity (including low birth weight, jaundice, retinopathy of prematurity, transfusions, surgery for removal of hemangenoma, and so forth) had and still have a profound impact on my life. Some people look at me and ask why I just cannot "get over it" and leave the prematurity and the NICU behind. I do not always know what to reply, but I know that for the rest of my life this experience will be with me, and I cannot ignore that it is happening to someone else, too.

BRAYDEN: THE STORY OF A FIGHTER

by Jayna Sattler

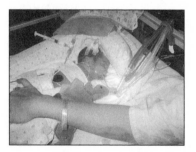 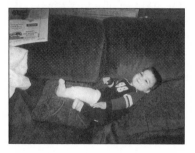

Brayden, two weeks old.   Brayden, sixteen months old.

The moment I found out I was pregnant I felt both elation and pure terror. After going through several pregnancy losses and a very high-risk pregnancy that ended in a premature baby boy, I felt that a normal pregnancy was impossible. I had no idea how right I was. We expected Brayden to be born just a little early due to his big brother's premature arrival, but what unfolded amazed and shocked me and my husband.

I found out I was pregnant just before Travis's first birthday, which was April 7, 1997. My pregnancy went as normally as can be expected for a high-risk pregnancy, except for a few bumps along the gestational journey. Our problems began when we lost a twin in the eighth week of pregnancy. I began having preterm contractions at nineteen weeks. I was put on terbutaline (a bronchodilator also used to inhibit premature labor) and bed rest. At twenty-two weeks I developed pneumonia from a severe case of bronchitis. I then began spotting and having contractions. Just a month after I recovered from the pneumonia, my water broke at twenty-eight weeks' gestation. I was rushed to the hospital, put on magnesium sulfate (a drug usually used to lower blood pressure but also used as a labor inhibitor), and transported to a larger hospital forty miles away that had a large Neonatal Intensive Care Unit (NICU). Three days later, when I was twenty-nine weeks pregnant, Brayden was born. My labor was fast and furious, and there was no stopping it since both the baby and I had developed an infection. Because I had so little amniotic fluid and my contractions were so intense, my uterus was literally crushing him. He went into distress, and the doctors began to contemplate a cesarean. They began an amnio-infusion, which eased his distress and allowed a vaginal delivery. He was born after only one hour and sixteen minutes of labor.

Brayden Thomas Sattler entered this world nearly three months early, on Friday, September 19, 1997, at 12:16 A.M., weighing 1,351 grams (2 pounds 15 ounces) and measuring 14 inches long. The doctors intubated him in the delivery room, and he was whisked away to the NICU. While he was not the smallest or sickest preemie ever to be born, we quickly learned that made little difference in his fight. He fought so hard to stay with us. After the delivery I was taken to my postpartum room to wait before seeing my precious bundle. I was greeted by another new mother who was nursing her healthy, chubby, full-term infant. I felt as if I had been stabbed in the back. I could do nothing but weep. This wasn't fair! I had done everything right to improve my chances of having a normal pregnancy and a healthy baby. Why did it go wrong?

The first time I saw my tiny son was on a TV screen in my postpartum room. There was a little red-skinned baby hooked up to so many tubes and wires that you could barely see him. There was also

a sign in his radiant warmer that read, "Hi, Mommy. I love you."
When my time was up for using the closed-circuit camera, the nurses
placed a sign that said, "I am very tired, Mommy. See you soon."
When I was allowed to visit him in person, they guided me into a
large washroom where they instructed me to scrub from my elbows
to my hands for three full minutes and then don a gown before entering the NICU. This was the first of my many, many scrub-ins.
After completing the scrub-in, I was escorted into the critical care
section of the unit. It was a very large and bright place with monitors beeping and ventilators humming and hissing. The room was
wall to wall with radiant warmers, each containing a tiny, sick infant. It was like another world. I walked over to a bed with a small
card identifying our son only as "Baby Boy Sattler—29 wks." It
seemed so impersonal. Didn't they know he had a name? I told the
nurse to please address him by his name, and soon she made a sign
with his name on it. I saw a beautiful baby boy who was so tiny and
scrawny that I likened him to a bird that had fallen out of his nest
much too soon. He had numerous IVs, a ventilator tube down his
throat, an umbilical catheter that ran to his heart, as well as monitor leads and probes all over his little body. As I watched the ventilator make his tiny chest rise and fall in rhythm, I could do nothing
but cry. What had I done wrong to make my child suffer so? Why
was this happening?

They soon told my husband and me exactly how sick our new son
was. He was septic with a strep infection, which ran rampant
throughout his body. His respiratory distress syndrome (RDS) was
worsening by the hour, and his oxygen requirements were increasing. We were informed later that they did not expect him to live more
than twenty-four hours. We refused to believe it. There was no way
we would let go of our tiny gift without a tremendous battle. He was
given two doses of Surfactant to help his small, immature lungs expand. I was released from the hospital only thirty-six hours after the
traumatic delivery. As they were wheeling me to the car, they put

me next to yet another new mother. She had her baby in her arms and was ready to take him home with her, where he belonged. My baby would remain in the NICU for the next two months, fighting for his life. I was leaving empty-handed and brokenhearted. I didn't even have as much as a new mom care pack. It was as if I hadn't delivered. We received no congratulations, cards, balloons, gifts—nothing.

On day three doctors discovered a grade I intraventricular hemorrhage (IVH) on the left side of Brayden's brain. We later learned that was only the beginning of his hemorrhaging. (In a later hospitalization they discovered that during the first week of life he had developed a grade III+ IVH in the right side.) After many tries and being put on Decadron (a steroid used to help wean him off the ventilator), he came off the ventilator for good sixteen days after his birth. He was still on oxygen and remained on it for twenty-two more days. He was on and off oxygen throughout the rest of his stay due to infections and pulmonary edema. Although his time on the ventilator was short, he developed bronchopulmonary dysplasia (BPD) and continues to fight with it. At two weeks of age they discovered that he had patent ductus arteriosus (PDA), so he was given indomethacin, and it closed without surgery.

Three weeks after his birth he graduated to a warmed isolette (also known as the Peanut Hut). Once he was able to maintain his body temperature a little better, we were introduced to kangaroo care. The nurses even encouraged his dad to participate in kangarooing. Brayden took to it like a fish to water. He seemed to love every second of being snuggled next to his mom or dad. At four weeks old he received his first feeding of breast milk via an oral gastric tube. Two weeks later he developed NEC (necrotizing enterocolitis) and had to be taken off oral feeds again. Fortunately, the NEC was caught early enough that he could recover with the help of antibiotics and bowel rest rather than surgery. He developed gastroesophageal reflux (GER) and was put on Reglan. He had an ongoing problem with anemia of prematurity and required more than the usual amount of blood transfusions. He had thirteen of them, to be exact.

I drew small posters that cheered Brayden on each week and taped them to his bed. We also taped pictures of us and his big brother for him to look at if he chose. We brought him stuffed animals to keep him company when we were away and to help personalize his space. I never missed visiting him a single day, although it meant an eighty-mile round trip. He had many, many battles with infections and numerous other setbacks, but after fifty-nine days in the NICU, on November 17, 1997, they released him to go home, weighing 5 pounds 4 ounces and measuring 17.5 inches. He was on no medication and no monitors. We thought everything was over, and we were finally going to become a normal family and have normal things happen.

Two weeks after his release, while I was holding him, he stopped breathing and had to be resuscitated. He was admitted to the pediatric intensive care unit (PICU) of his birth hospital. It was found that he still had severe central apnea and bradycardia, along with GER. He was also in anemic crisis and was given a double blood transfusion that night. He was placed on theophylline, Reglan, and a home monitor. The doctors sent him home a week later. He continued to have severe episodes, many to the point of arrest. We have resuscitated him more times than we care to count. They later diagnosed him with reactive airway disorder (RAD) due to scarring from being intubated and extubated, along with the gavage feedings, so albuterol nebulizer treatments were also added to his cocktail of medications. He was also put on Propulsid in addition to the Reglan for his reflux. He entered the Early Intervention program after his second homecoming.

At five months of age he fell ill again. As I was driving him to the local ER for a respiratory synctial virus (RSV) culture, he arrested. When I arrived at the ER, he was in complete arrest. As I placed him on the gurney in the trauma room, I thought I was laying down a dead baby. They started CPR immediately. He revived quickly and was admitted. An EKG was run to rule out cardiac involvement, which they soon dismissed when it was normal. They transferred him to his birth hospital and admitted him to the PICU again. He did have an upper respiratory infection, but it was not RSV. He also had gastric inflammation and sepsis. An EEG and MRI of the brain were run two days later. The EEG was normal, showing no evidence of seizure activity. The MRI, on the other hand, was anything but normal. It showed generalized atrophy of the brain, excessive cerebral-spinal fluid, an enlarged left ventricle, and significant damage to the right side, the result of a grade III or higher hemorrhage suffered in the first weeks of life. As the neurologist pointed out each area of damage, I choked back tears. I wanted to scream that he was wrong, it was not Brayden's film, it was all a mistake. I knew in my heart they had made no mistake, but I couldn't believe my little baby would still have such a fight ahead of him.

We left the hospital more frustrated and frightened than before. What did life hold for Brayden? Would he have any normalcy to him at all? His official diagnosis then was recurring apparent life-threatening event (ALTE), tightening of the airway causing wheezing (RAD), and neurological damage. After another week in the hospital and many tests later, we left feeling more hopeless and helpless than ever before.

As things continue to progress, he has been diagnosed with spastic quadriplegic cerebral palsy, epilepsy, cortical blindness to the right field of vision, strabismus, amblyopia, nystagmus, severe and prolonged bradycardia with apnea, failure to thrive, and oral defensiveness. He also has been diagnosed with craniosynostosis (premature fusion on the fontanels). He currently receives physical therapy twice a week and occupational/speech therapy once a week. Brayden has also begun hippotherapy, which is horseback riding coupled with physical therapy. He is progressing better than expected, but there is still a long and difficult journey ahead.

At eighteen months old, Brayden continues to fight each day. He amazes us with his perseverance and strength. He will beat the odds!

RYAN'S STORY: A LIFE FULL OF MIRACLES

by Robin White

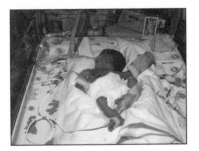

Ryan, three days old.

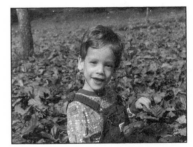

Ryan, two years old.

When I learned I was pregnant with our second child, I was both happy and worried. Due to placenta previa, my first pregnancy had several complications. Our oldest son, Travis, almost came seven weeks early, but doctors were able to hold off labor for five more weeks. The first few months of the second pregnancy were going pretty well. The morning sickness that was so awful with the first pregnancy was not as bad this time, and so far there were no signs of previa. Then into the last part of my third month it started. I was rushed to the emergency room, where the doctors told me they were worried about a miscarriage. The bleeding stopped, and I was sent home to do as much resting as I could, but when you have a two-year-old, that is not so easy. I was thankful my sister came to help because although I was not on complete bed rest, the less I did, the better.

During this time my father had been fighting a battle with cancer. We lived in Texas, and my parents lived a little over five hundred miles away in Mississippi. When my husband, who was in the Air Force, was sent to Japan for a month, it was decided that our son and I would go for a visit. I hadn't seen my husband in a while and thought the visit with our son might do him good. I was six months along at this time. Little did I know that we would not be heading to Japan.

We had been visiting my parents for about two weeks when suddenly my dad passed away. Needless to say, I was devastated, and the stress over the next couple of days would take its toll. Thank goodness that with the help of the Red Cross my husband was able to return to the United States.

The day after the funeral I started having small pains in the lower part of my stomach, but it was not like contractions, so I didn't think I was in labor. We decided to go to the emergency room. The doctor told me I was having contractions, but they were very small, I was not in labor, and it would be a good idea for me to return to our home in Texas as soon as possible so my doctor could check me out. The next morning we started back home. I hated leaving my mom and sisters, but to be on the safe side I needed to be close to my doctor. We were only three hours into the trip when the pains began increasing. We had stopped at a visitor's center when the first "real" contraction started. We were told the next town with a hospital was approximately sixty miles away. We had been through this town a number of times but didn't know anything about its hospitals. My husband went as fast as he could, and my pains continued to increase. I began to worry about making it to the hospital in time.

When we arrived in this Louisiana town, my husband followed the signs to the hospital. I was rushed in, and my husband, who was holding our very confused two-year-old, was running behind us. The doctor said that I was definitely in labor, and she would do all she could to stop it. Upon examination it was determined I was too far into labor, and I would be giving birth at any moment. My husband was called into my room. (I found out later that the nurses at the front desk had been taking care of Travis.) The neonatologist arrived and explained to us what would happen as soon as the baby was born. We were scared to death. I had just lost my father, and now I might lose my baby. This had to be a dream.

An hour after arriving at the hospital Ryan Houston was born, weighing 2 pounds 10 ounces. All I could do was pray as they were working with him. The cord had prolapsed, and he was barely breathing. After what seemed like forever, the doctors were able to stabilize him, and he was immediately intubated. All I saw of Ryan was the back of his tiny head as they rushed him out. It would be several hours before we were able to see him.

We weren't sure what to expect in the NICU. As we entered, it was such a shock, with several rows of beds containing the smallest babies we had ever seen. They were hooked up to so many tubes and wires that you had to look very hard just to see the babies. I was thinking, "Dear God, is this what my baby looks like?" When we reached his bed, I learned that he did. Here lay our son Ryan, tiny and helpless.

The neonatologist proceeded to update us on his condition. At this point it did not look good. His lungs were in horrible shape. He was under a bilirubin light because he was jaundiced. He was purple-looking and very swollen with fluid because of his quick birth. There were so many medical terms and so many machines being explained that my head was spinning. I never imagined that after being there for a while I would be able to tell others these terms, exactly what each machine was, and what every beep and bell meant!

Our two-year-old went to stay with my mom and sisters. I was worried about this since it had been only a few days after my mom had lost her husband of twenty-five years. But my sisters felt it would be just what she needed. My husband was able to stay a few days but had to report back to the base after a while. I spent the next seven weeks at a house nearby that was for family members with loved ones in the hospital. It was the greatest place. The lady who ran the house became my greatest source of support when my husband and family were not there.

Every day started the same—going straight to the hospital to see Ryan. First the questions: How is he? Did he have a good night? How is his weight? The nurses answered my questions the best they could, and the doctor filled me in on the rest. The matter of transferring Ryan to our hometown came up over and over, but it would not be an option for some time. His lungs were in pretty bad shape. One side had started to collapse at one point and a chest tube was inserted. It was also discovered that he had a grade 3 IVH. Before my husband left he had been asked to give blood for Ryan because they had taken so much to have it tested for infections and also for doing blood gases. Ryan would need more blood after a while, and my husband would have to drive four hours to donate because he was in one state and Ryan in another.

I was not in the best shape myself, either emotionally or physically. I cried constantly, especially if I heard another baby cry or if I saw a healthy baby. I soon found an alternate route to the NICU because the other way passed right by the nursery. My breaking point came the day before I was released. I was in the bathroom and heard a mother in the next room singing to her baby. I lost it. My husband tried to console me, but it just hurt too much. It was not fair. My son lay in the NICU, hooked up to so many wires and tubes that I could not hold him, and here she was singing and rocking her baby. I soon realized that if I was going to get through this and stay somewhat sane, I was going to have to get a grip on things, so I started pumping breast milk. Even though Ryan could not have it at this time, I knew he would soon need it, and I wanted to have it ready. I would sit and talk to Ryan. I also sang to him and held his tiny hand. I wanted Ryan to know I was there for him.

Then one day I wasn't feeling well. I was running a high fever and felt weak. I went to the doctor and discovered I had a kidney infection. I was hospitalized that day. This could not be happening! I couldn't be sick! I was hospitalized for only a couple of days, but it seemed like forever. Because of the medication I was on, my milk soon stopped, and I had to quit pumping. I was so upset. I felt I was letting Ryan down. The nurses assured me that the milk I had already saved would be a great help to Ryan.

Finally, the day we had been waiting for arrived: Ryan could be transferred. He was still critical, but he could be transferred back to Texas. This process turned into a nightmare. The insurance company at first did not want to do it, but with a doctor's urging the go-ahead was given. Our family would finally be in one state! I packed up, hugged all the nurses, and thanked the doctors at least a million times.

For the next two months Ryan would remain on the ventilator. Several attempts to take him off were made but failed. He could not handle it. Visiting the hospital every day was now our routine. I spent as much time as I could with Ryan, but I also had to think of the child at home. I planned "special times" just for Travis. We would go for ice cream or to the zoo. I always made sure I was home to put him in bed at night and read him a story. I did not want him to feel forgotten in all this.

I questioned a nurse one day about holding Ryan. She was shocked to learn that it had been seven weeks and I had not held him. With him on the ventilator, the doctor was not comfortable with his being held. The nurse talked to Ryan's new doctor, and I was able to hold Ryan for just a minute. All I could do was cry. It was the best feeling in the world.

One of Ryan's many surgeries came when he reached three

months old. He needed hernia surgery, and it was also determined that he needed surgery on his eyes. He had grade 3 ROP. Both surgeries would be done at the same time. Ryan was moved to the children's hospital across the street. He stayed there for the next six weeks. The pulmonologist explained to us about Ryan's lungs. She said that with BPD it was hard to determine how long recovery would take.

Ryan's condition was getting better, but he wasn't taking the bottle the way the doctors thought he should. When Ryan was given his first bottle, he did not do very well. He wore out too quickly. He was fed a while longer through a tube in his nose. Each day we tried it, again and again. He was tested, and it was determined that after being on the ventilator for so long, he had a very narrow airway. With the BPD and his airway so small, he would give out after just a few seconds with the bottle. Another test was done, and we discovered that Ryan had reflux. With this and his inability to take a bottle, it was decided that a g-button (tube inserted in the belly button) and fundoplication (when the top of the stomach is fixed so the reflux cannot go back into the esophagus) would be done. We would be able to feed Ryan through the g-button until he was able to take a bottle himself. Poor baby, all he had been through and now a feeding tube. What next?

Waiting during this surgery seemed like a lifetime. I was so worried. He was still so tiny. The surgery went well except that problems arose with the incision. It opened up and made a very nasty-looking wound. The doctors believe this was from the steroids Ryan had been on.

Learning to use the g-button did not take long. It was scary at first, but after a while we got the hang of it and talk of coming home came up. It had been four long months! Even though Ryan's lungs were still weak from the BPD, it was determined that he could go home. He would be on breathing treatments with a nebulizer. We were taught how to do this and were given CPR classes.

After we were trained in CPR and were shown how to do all of Ryan's care, we did our "rooming in." This is when the parents spend one night at the hospital so that if any problems occur, a nurse is there to help. Needless to say, we did not sleep a wink. Ryan went home on an apnea monitor and had to receive nebulizer treatments, tube feedings, and wound care on his stomach from where his incision opened up. A home health nurse was to come by once a week to check on this and make sure it was healing properly.

The big day finally came. It had been four months. My mom came out to help, and our two-year-old was very excited about "baby brudder" coming home. He had seen Ryan in the NICU, but it was hard to explain why his brother was there at first. After he saw him and saw his "boo-boos," he understood. I don't think we slept the first few months Ryan was home—with feedings every three hours, constant monitor beeps, and just getting up in general to make sure everything was okay.

Ryan was such a happy baby. He smiled all the time (a smile the size of Texas) and had the best disposition. The doctors were amazed. I was told preemies were usually cranky and did not sleep very well. Ryan slept the entire night the first night he was home and has done so until just a couple of months ago.

Because of Ryan's long stay in the hospital and his surgeries, his muscles did not develop as they should have. He had very weak muscle tone. Ryan also had an aversion to anything going into his mouth, so at around six months he started speech and physical therapy. Like a lot of preemies, Ryan started late on everything. His first word was not until he was one year old, and it was "bye-bye," the best word I have ever heard! He started trying to sit up at twenty months and was doing it well by twenty-four months. He is still working on walking. He does crawl and can climb like a squirrel.

Ryan's first eighteen months were filled with doctors' appointments, therapy sessions, and several hospital stays due to respiratory problems. The first winter it seemed he caught everything around even though we kept him away from everybody. In January he contracted RSV. He spent almost a month in the hospital this time—two weeks of that in isolation in the PICU. During this time he also needed a chest tube inserted because his lung had partially collapsed. What amazed the doctors was that he did not have to be intubated even though his airway was still small and his lungs were in bad shape. This was truly a miracle—or should I say just one of the many miracles we have encountered during all this.

In April 1997, Ryan was having trouble with retching and gagging when I would tube-feed him. With suggestions from the doctors and nutritionist, we tried everything from slowing the feedings down to splitting them up. Nothing worked. Finally, after some tests, it was discovered that Ryan had a hernia in his diaphragm. At first it was believed to be a congenital diaphragmatic hernia (CDH), which means this was something he could have had since birth and was just now showing up. It was also decided at this time to check his airway. The doctors had hoped that as Ryan grew, so would his airway. Ryan had been doing so well, and we thought all the surgeries and problems were finally over. The results from the surgery were of the good news, bad news kind. Good news: It was not a CDH, just a hernia in the diaphragm, and was repairable. Bad news: Ryan's airway had not grown. In fact, the narrowing seemed to go farther down than first thought. The surgeon had told us he would do a procedure to try to dilate the airway with a "balloon" in hopes of opening the airway. It had not worked yet, so another surgery was scheduled. "This could not be happening," I thought. "Dear Lord, why?"

It would be two weeks before the next surgery could be done because, first, they had to let the surgery for the hernia heal. Second, Ryan's lungs had developed and filled with mucus. Ryan had been left intubated after the surgery. His airway was swollen too badly to be taken off.

The day before the next surgery, the surgeon explained to us what would happen. The surgery would take two to three hours. Ryan would be sedated for two more weeks so he would be still to let the incision heal. He would also need to be intubated during this time. That broke my heart. It was the very thing that caused all this. There were no guarantees that this procedure would work. Ryan could still have problems. One concern was whether he would be able to talk; another, that he might need a trach. So we waited yet again. We geared ourselves up for the two- or three-hour wait. Could I get through this without going nuts?

We had been in the waiting room for about forty-five minutes when the surgeon came in. I did not know whether to faint or sit there. I asked what he was doing there, and he said, "We're done!" What? It seems the narrowing was not as bad as first thought. They were able to do a procedure that was not as involved as the one they were prepared to do. Ryan was not going to need a trach, and his voice should be fine!

The next two weeks were long ones. Ryan's incision was healing nicely. He did have some lung problems, but they seemed to be improving. Then the big day came. It was time to get the tube out. He had failed to come off the ventilator after the first surgery, and I was very nervous about this time. The PICU was quiet. Everyone was watching. I couldn't stop crying. Ryan was doing great. He was still groggy from all the medication he had been on, but he was breathing wonderfully! I held him for two hours. I didn't want to let him go.

After a few days he was ready to go home. It would take a few weeks for the medications to wear off and for him to get back to his old self. When he did, he came back with a bang! His breathing was great, his lungs were wonderful, and he started babbling. Everything he had not been doing before the surgery he was trying now. He was even putting things to his mouth, something he had never done. He just kept doing better and better after that. His eating improved immensely. We also had fewer doctors' appointments. What a relief that was!

Ryan is now two and a half years old and doing wonderfully. He truly has amazed everyone. He is eating and drinking and gaining weight. So his g-button came out. We no longer see the speech therapist. His talking is great, and he loves to tell knock-knock jokes that his older brother teaches him. He gets around but doesn't walk independently. He's also a Barney and Elmo fan.

Doctors believe some of his problems stem from the IVH but in time he will catch up with his peers. His breathing treatments will stop soon. He had a great winter—his only hospital stay was for a mild case of pneumonia, and that was only overnight. His pulmonologist is thrilled with his development and the way his lungs have healed. He is doing better than anyone ever thought possible.

My husband and I have learned a lot about ourselves. We are stronger people, and we cherish every day with our children. We have learned that life is too precious to be in a hurry or to worry about little things. We have a friendship now with some of the other parents from the NICU and PICU. I think it is because we can understand what the others are going through, and if we need someone to talk to, we can call each other. I guess you can say we have our own little support system.

Ryan has been through a lot in his two and a half years, but he has made it and is doing great. If I were to give any advice to other parents of preemies, it would be: Never give up hope!

OUR LITTLE PICKLE:
GRIFFIN'S STORY

by Karen Cork

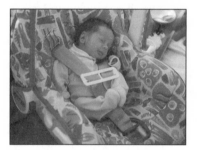

Griffin, twenty-one days old.

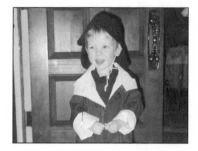

Griffin, twenty-five months old.

I was fourteen weeks pregnant when I discovered thin pink blood upon wiping. I immediately fell apart and panicked, sure that I was going to lose this baby I had wanted all my life. I had expected that if anything were going to go wrong, it would happen in the first twelve weeks; that is what everyone always said. After three months you are home free.

My husband took me to the emergency room. I was given an internal exam, but the doctor said he was going easy on it since he did not want to disturb the placenta if it was low lying. A strong and healthy heartbeat was detected, the baby was not in distress. Many "possibles" came out of the doctor's mouth: "possible late miscarriage," "possible cervix irritation," and "possible placenta previa." I knew what placenta previa was but not what it meant for me and my baby. The next day I went for an ultrasound, and the PP was confirmed; in addition, my placenta was completely covering the cervical opening. I was instructed to stop having sex (intercourse and orgasms) for the duration of the pregnancy. I was also told, "No excercise of any kind, not even brisk walks."

From what I understand from my doctors, usually the placenta attaches itself to the top side of the uterus. With PP it attaches itself at the bottom, a part of the uterus that is not meant for this kind of demand. The bottom of the uterus changes shape, stretches, and expands throughout a pregnancy, preparing for the growth of the baby and for the baby to move down as delivery approaches. The placenta can lift or tear away from the uterus during these shape changes, causing bleeding. The placenta is the life force for the baby, where blood and nutrients move from the mother's body to the baby's, but any bleeding is the mother's blood, not the baby's. When the doctor told me this, I felt much better.

My doctor said that 90 percent of pregnancies begin with a low placenta and that usually by twenty-eight weeks the placenta has found its way back up near the top of the uterus where it should be. (I should point out that I thought this meant the placenta would move, but it actually means that as the uterus grows and expands, the placenta "appears" to move upwards; it does not actually move but follows the shifting of the uterus.) If this was not the case with me, I should expect a cesarean section delivery since a vaginal delivery would be impossible, risking my life and the baby's. My next ultrasound was scheduled for twenty-eight to thirty weeks. During this time I was not given an internal exam, and all pressure on the fundus was limited to the top, with very little poking and prodding near the bottom so as not to disturb the placenta.

The Second Bleed

My pregnancy after that was without further incident. I continued work (acting and teaching drama to children, light housework, no lifting, and so forth) until twenty-three weeks when, after no exertion whatsoever, I stood up from my chair and felt blood gush. I knew that blood could come at any time, that there was no need to think I had done anything to cause bleeding. This gush was as much blood as a heavy first day of a period.

Kevin, my hubby, drove me to the hospital about twenty minutes away in about ten minutes. They rushed me to labor and delivery. (Although I did not know this at the time, they took me right to this ward because they thought I was going to deliver—a precaution in order to be ready for an emergency C-section.) My blood was typed in case I needed a transfusion (not needed). I was put on an IV drip. An ultrasound showed that the placenta was running down one side of my uterus, across the cervix, and growing back up the other side. The baby was in no distress and growing at a normal speed. The nurses told me, however, that if the baby were born now, at twenty-three weeks, there would not be a lot they could do for him. Right now they were concerned with my health and blood loss. Since arriving at the hospital I had felt four gushes, the last two being described by the nurse as "nothing at all, not to worry!" I was given a shot of steroids to help the baby's lungs to mature faster, although the doctors said that at twenty-three weeks it might be too early for them to make a difference.

After two hours I stopped bleeding entirely but was still confined to total bed rest, with bed pan use only. I was admitted overnight because they do not release PP patients until they have stopped bleeding for twenty-four hours. In the morning I was able to get up and go to the washroom, where I panicked again at the site of a brown discharge. I was told it was the old blood from the episode clearing itself out. I was released twenty-four hours after admission with instructions from the doctor on call: "No sex, no exercise, bed rest as much as possible, no lifting, no sneezing or coughing." (I was to take a powerful cough medicine to prevent a bad cough.) I found out later from my OB-GYN that these were extreme instructions; however, it was not hard to avoid sneezing for the rest of my pregnancy, and although it probably would not have made any difference, it made me feel better. I was also told to keep my bowel movements regular and soft, because straining would also threaten the placenta. In hindsight, this on-call doctor in the hospital may have leaned too far on the side of caution (all my other doctors agree). My own doctor told me to go ahead and keep working. I chose to err on the side of caution and quit my job, restrained all sneezes (for nine solid weeks!), and spent a lot of time lying down.

After my discharge from the hospital, I was referred to an OB-GYN, a specialist who had a lot of experience with PP. He was a little less cautious, warning only against sex and exercise, but he did drop two bombshells. First, I would have to be admitted to the hospital at thirty-two weeks for the duration of the pregnancy since the risk of bleeding becomes greater then. Apparently the uterus begins to expand at the bottom, increasing the chance that the placenta will pull away from the uterine wall. I would be in the hospital under observation in case I began to bleed again. According to this doctor, the bleeds would get worse each time, so I should expect it and not freak out; it was all part of the placenta previa. I prepared for a four- to six-week stay in the hospital. This doctor planned to do an amniocentesis at thirty-five weeks, and as soon as the baby's lungs were mature, he would perform the C-section. Second, there was the remote chance that the placenta would grow into the uterine wall, making it impossible to deliver or remove, causing life-threatening bleeding. The only option if this occurred was a hysterectomy. He assured me that this would be a last resort and would be done only to save my life. In his career he had had to do this only once. I was asked to sign a release form stating that I gave permission to perform the hysterectomy "if my life depended on it." I knew I could accept this occurrence only if the baby in my womb survived.

The Third Bleed

Again, there were no episodes until twenty-nine weeks, and then a thin pinky wipe meant another trip to the hospital, another admission, and all the same precautions as before. This time the staff was positive about my baby's chances if born now. This bleed was not as bad as the twenty-third week one (never a gush, only the one wipe), and none of us really expected the baby to come. All monitors and ultrasounds showed the baby was fine and the placenta was still down south. I was given a second shot of steroids for the baby's lungs. I had received the first shot at twenty-three weeks, but at that time the doctor thought it was too early to make a difference. I was discharged again the next day after no bleeding. Home again and on the couch, cooking the baby.

At thirty weeks and three days I found "old brown" blood on a wipe. This did not scare me nearly as much. My husband and I were on the way to the hospital for prenatal classes, and I dropped in to tell the nurses on the predelivery ward what had happened (a place I had come to know all too well by now). They surprised me by saying they thought it was enough to admit me again. Another shot of steroids. This time I did not get to go home.

My OB-GYN came in the next morning and said that three bleeds were just too many for him to feel comfortable sending me home. He wanted me in the hospital for the duration. To tell the truth, I was relieved. I never relaxed at home, worrying about the possibility of another big bleed when Kevin was out or not getting to the hospital on time. Going into the hospital for what I thought was going to be five or six weeks was not difficult for me. I had quit my job and had no other children at home. I was given passes to go to restaurants or movie theaters across the street from the hospital. On Saturday, June 8, the doctor on call gave me a tour of the NICU and the operating room.

On Sunday, June 9, I had brown spotting and was put on bed rest again. Until now I could visit my new PP friend, Monica, in her room, go for walks around the ward, stroll to the nursery and the TV room, and have three-hour passes to go across the street. Now I was in bed. I remember worrying out loud to a nurse: "What if I started the big bleed in the middle of the night?" She said, "Oh, don't worry, you will wake up. That is one thing about being pregnant—you know that you are not supposed to bleed, so when you do, you notice it!" Funny we should have this conversation because at 6 A.M. on Monday, June 10, I woke up feeling a gush and buzzed the nurse. She came immediately with Maalox (I had wicked heartburn and asked for it at least every four to six hours, so she made a natural assumption), but, alas, this was not a heartburn issue. A sudden flurry of activity, fetal monitors, some medicine that I cannot remember the name of to calm down my slightly growing contractions—a complete weird major allergic reaction! Suddenly I could not keep my eyes open. Everyone in the room seemed to be miles away. I was slurring my words. My blood pressure was low, and I was sooooooo dizzy although I was lying down. In the event of surgery I could have nothing to eat or drink—not even Maalox!

Another shot of steroids, but who knows if they made any difference. I am going to be a bit more graphic now. This bleed was a gush about every three minutes or so—enough to soak a pad in less than an hour. I mention this because it was something my doctor focused on a lot when we discussed how much blood there had been in my previous episodes. Apparently he worried only when you could soak a pad in under an hour.

My bleeding quit at about 1 P.M. for at least a few hours. The nurses then allowed me to eat three glorious wedges of watermelon from the gods before I started bleeding again, around 3 P.M. By 6 my baby's heart rate was too fast. I did not know that this was dangerous, too. I thought only a low heart rate was worrisome. At a few minutes past six on the first day of my thirty-second week of pregnancy the decision was made to do an emergency C-section. There was a bigger flurry of activity. Signing forms that authorized the doctor to perform a hysterectomy if I didn't stop bleeding was the hardest part (thankfully, this never had to happen). Catheters and IVs were inserted, and blood pressure finger monitors were attached. My darling hubby, who had come in the morning, left when I quit bleeding but rushed right back when I started again. Suddenly he was making frantic phone calls to family members, all the while being instructed on how to get into scrubs and wash up. Bless his heart, through the window of the operating room while he was changing he made faces at me to make me giggle and relax.

C-Section Time

Now let me tell you. I was not concerned about having a C-section. Heck, they could have ripped Griffin out my left nostril, and I wouldn't have cared as long as he was okay. I know there are many women who are sad not to have a "normal" birth. My first bit of advice: Change the word "normal" to "vaginal." You are spared the contraction pain but make up for it in major surgery pain during the recovery afterward, and otherwise there are not many differences. I was able to be awake for the birth (this may not always be the case depending on the seriousness of the bleed). At the moment they brought Griffin out of my womb, they dropped the surgical screen so that Kevin and I could see Griffin being born. It is true that I have not experienced a vaginal birth, but I cannot imagine that the joy of seeing your baby born that way is any greater than what I felt at that moment.

My Preemie Baby

Griffin was big, so wonderfully big, and he cried right away—and so did I. I was expecting a 3½- to 4-pound baby. Griffin was 5 pounds exactly. He scored 9 on both Apgars. He was breathing on his own. This may have been due to the steroids I received (three shots over ten weeks) or, as I read in *What to Expect the First Year* by Arlene Eisenberg, Heidi E. Murkoff, and Sandee E. Hathaway, "babies who have undergone severe stress in the uterus, usually during labor and delivery, are less likely to lack surfactants (a detergent-like substance that gives the lung surfaces their elastic properties) as the stress appears to speed lung maturation."

I could not hold Griffin right away since he had to be rushed to the NICU, but Kevin held him up to me and I touched his wee cheek. I am bawling my eyes out at this moment remembering. I held him for the first time at eleven hours old. He was in an incubator on oxygen with an IV in his head (a precaution for possible infection, they told me).

On Griffin's second day of life he started to go backward. There was talk of transferring him to a larger hospital and venting his lungs to add some surfactants, but after two days (during which we could not hold him) on his back with an IV in his umbilical cord to monitor blood gases, he proved everyone wrong and turned around. He has been like this all his life. Every time I begin to worry about anything, he immediately does or does not do whatever it was I was pulling my hair out about.

When Griffin was six days old, they removed his IV. On day seven he graduated to the bassinet and room air. I tried breast-feeding on day four; it went slowly. He could not stay awake since all his energy was spent working those little lungs. He nursed every second feed but was tube-fed every other one to make sure he got a proper meal to build up his strength.

On day 21, June 30, 1996, my darling pickle came home to his father and me. He has me wrapped around his tiny little finger, and there is nowhere else I would rather be.

LESSONS FROM A CHILD:
NOAH'S STORY

by Jan Sweeney

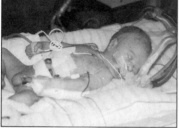

Noah, one week old.

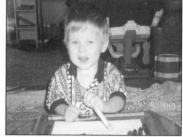

Noah, three years old.

Noah Patrick Sweeney missed out on the last two months in utero. Noah also has VACTERLS syndrome, a group of birth defects not related to prematurity. Noah's story is one of a child with an extreme will to live. I have said many times that there is no reason that Noah should be alive today. Most babies who have as many birth defects as Noah are miscarried. Noah had the added challenge of being premature. It is hard to say which of Noah's problems are from being premature and which of his problems are from VACTERLS. All his problems are complicated by the others.

Noah's story began in September 1994. My husband had been adamant about not having a baby. He was afraid that something would happen to me. I tried to convince him that hardly anyone dies in childbirth anymore. Finally, one day out of the blue, he said that maybe it was time to try to have a baby. I was ecstatic because I had been waiting to hear that for months. Brian and I had been married for two years and had just bought a house in a small town in Wyoming. Our life was on track, and it was time to add to our family. I went to the doctor, got a checkup, and stopped taking the pill. My doctor told me that everything should go well. I was only twenty-two years old and very healthy. I did everything I could to ensure that we would have a healthy baby. I stopped drinking caffeine, did not smoke or drink alcohol, and began eating right.

Six months later I found out I was pregnant. I was on top of the world. All my husband could say was "How?" When it hit him that he was going to be a daddy, he was so proud. Later that day I went to the doctor to confirm the pregnancy and found my baby was due on Christmas Day. Once again the doctor said everything looked good, and it should be a routine pregnancy—and it was, for a while. Other than morning sickness, I felt great. I did not gain much weight until I was about five months along. My first ultrasound, at eighteen weeks, was, as the doctor put it, questionable. They did not see everything they had hoped to see and so wanted to repeat it in a few weeks. I was told that the baby was probably in a weird position. At the second ultrasound four weeks later, I was told that my baby was a boy. He got a clean bill of health. They said they did not see a stomach bubble, but that was not unusual for his gestational age. So I went about my business being a happy, relatively healthy pregnant lady. I did the normal things that pregnant mommies do: bought a crib, car seat, and thousands of baby things (okay, maybe not thousands!).

At my thirty-one-week checkup the doctor was very concerned that my blood pressure was high. I had gained about 20 pounds since my last visit and developed carpal tunnel syndrome. I was working only about three or four hours a day, so he knew that the carpal tunnel was not from excessive typing. Since I may have been developing preeclampsia, the doctor ordered strict bed rest for a week. I was pretty faithful about the bed rest until the next weekend. I just couldn't take it anymore; I had to get out. I went with some friends to a town about forty miles away to do some Christmas shopping. After all, in a few months I knew I would not feel like shopping. The next day we decided to go to Denver, Colorado, to look at a car with my in-laws. I felt really good all day and tried to lounge in the car. It was a fun weekend. In retrospect, however, I know that I should have stayed home. Nothing I did would have changed anything, though; it would have just postponed it.

The next day, Monday, at my appointment my blood pressure was through the roof. I had gained even more weight. The doctor put me in the hospital immediately. They did blood work on me and a stress test on the baby. I thought that I would be in and out the next day and so was not too concerned, but I was nervous because I did not know what to expect. The thought of having a preemie did not even occur to me. The stress test showed that the baby was doing great. The next morning the doctor came in to check on me. He had just gotten some test results back and told me I was very sick. My kidneys had almost completely shut down, and my liver was well on its way. He had already called a hospital in Denver, and they were sending Life Flight to pick me up. I was absolutely terrified. I asked my doctor how long the baby and I would be in the hospital. He told me that the baby probably weighed about 5 pounds, and we should be in the hospital about a week. How could this be happening to us? I was young and healthy, I had never been in the hospital before, and now they were flying me to a hospital in Denver. It was almost like a dream, and the drugs the doctor put me on did not help that feeling. It was as though someone had taken my perfect little snow globe life and shaken it so hard that the snow would never stop falling.

When I arrived in Denver, they immediately took me to have an ultrasound and an amniocentesis to see if the baby's lungs were developed enough to be born. At this point they were very concerned about my health. I was put on magnesium sulfate to lower my blood pressure, which made me feel awful and completely out of it. I hardly remember being in the hospital. I knew my family was with me, and they were very nervous. I was terrified.

I was not getting any better; I was getting worse. The only thing that would help me get better was having the baby, so they wanted to deliver him as soon as possible. During the ultrasound, the doctor found that once again the baby had no stomach bubble. I mentioned that they did not see one in the previous ultrasound, which told the doctor immediately that we had a problem. The baby had a condition called esophageal atresia—essentially there was no esophagus. They continued to look and soon found cardiac defects. As we were finishing the ultrasound, the doctor explained to my husband and me that our baby was about to be born two months too soon, seriously underweight for his gestational age, and with serious birth defects, probably Down's syndrome. It seemed as though he had three strikes against him before he was even born. All I could think about was, why me, why us? Looking back, my thoughts were more about how this would affect me rather than how my child would be affected. I was very young to deal with things like this. More than young, I think I was very immature. But being put in this situation forces you to grow up very quickly. I know I am a very different person now than when my son was born, but I knew then that I would love him and take care of him no matter what.

The amniocentesis confirmed that the baby was not ready to be born. My new perinatologist (maternal fetal medicine specialist) wanted me to stay pregnant as long as I could. They were giving me steroids to mature the baby's lungs more quickly. A neonatal cardiologist was brought in to do a cardiac ultrasound on the baby. It was confirmed that he had a hole between the upper two chambers of his heart, or an atrial septal defect. There was nothing we could do until after he was born. The next day the focus came off the baby's problems and on mine. The doctors were very concerned that I was going to have a stroke or that my liver would rupture. Because they wanted to give the baby a little more time inside me, it was decided that they would induce labor early the next morning. I was terrified. I remember asking one of the nurses if I was going to die. Doctors from the NICU came in to tell us what to expect when the baby was born. That was just as scary. I was afraid that I would not get to see my baby. I was afraid he would die. The doctors were not being very optimistic about his chances. I had never seen a premature baby, and the picture they painted was not a pretty one. I could not imagine how he would look or that he would be strong enough to fight the battle he had to fight.

Early the next morning, at about 4 o'clock, they began inducing labor. Everything went according to plan, and at 10:59 P.M., on November 9, 1995, Noah Patrick Sweeney made his entrance, weighing 1,660 grams (3 pounds 10 ounces) and 17¾ inches long. I was so out of it by the time he was born that I just told them to take him and fix him. I remember seeing a tiny blue leg as he was passed to the NICU respiratory therapist. There seemed to be about fifty people in the room all rushing to save my baby. I did hear the tiniest of cries—the most wonderful sound I had ever heard. The neonatologist did not think Noah would be able to cry due to his immature lungs. Remember that girl who I said was more worried about how a disabled child would affect her? Well, at 10:59 P.M. she left. As soon as I heard that little cry, I knew that I would do whatever was necessary to make sure that that tiny boy would have the best life possible. I knew at that moment all that mattered was that little man.

Shortly after Noah was born, I think I passed out. I was so full of drugs and so exhausted that I had to sleep. I vaguely remember the surgeon and neonatologist coming in at about 1 A.M. to tell us about Noah's problems and about the surgery he was about to undergo. Fortunately, he did not have Down's syndrome. However, Noah was born with VACTERLS syndrome. Each letter stands for a birth defect:

- Vertebrae: He has three malformed vertebrae, scoliosis, three extra ribs, and his ribs are very thin.
- Anus: Noah was born without an anus. The first surgery that the surgeon performed was to form a colostomy.
- Cardiac: Noah had an atrial septal defect.
- TE for trachoesphageal fistula: Noah's trachea was connected to his esophagus. In the first surgery they were also going to disconnect his trachea from his esophagus and put a tube directly into his stomach so he could eat.
- Renal: Noah was born with only one kidney.
- Limb: Noah had no limb defects. Most kids with VACTERLS have serious limb defects.
- Single umbilical artery: Noah only had one umbilical artery.

Noah went to surgery when he was just four hours old. He did very well and came out on a ventilator and very stable. The next morning I was too sick to see him. It killed me that I could not hold my little man and let him know that it would be all right. My son needed me, his mother. I was his mother, and my job from that point forward was to protect and love my son. I did not know how hard it would be to protect my son, though. I guess you could say I was about to get a crash course in motherhood. It was weird to think of myself as a mother. My mom and dad had always been there making decisions for me, and now I was the one responsible for this little helpless person. I was now the one who would be making the decisions. At that time I did not realize that I would literally be making life-and-death decisions for my son.

Finally, when Noah was about thirty-six hours old, they allowed me to see him. I had seen a video and pictures of him, but nothing could prepare me for what I was about to see. There was hardly a baby there at all—just this tiny bird without feathers and with tubes all over his body. When I touched him, these big blue eyes looked up at me as if he already knew I was his mother. A mat of blond curly hair covered a tiny head that looked as if it would crush under the weight of my hand. The nurse was trying to explain all the machines to me, but all I could think about was how badly I wanted to take him away from all this. This was not how it was supposed to happen. I knew that at any moment I would wake up and my son would be in bed with me nursing. He was far too tiny and fragile to endure the things he had and the things I knew he was up against. I was able to stay with him for only a very short time. I still had a lot of recuperating to do, and so did my little man.

I snuck down to the NICU every chance I could the next day and stayed a little while each time. All I could do was sit and stare at him and touch his tiny hands. It was amazing to me that this was my son. I also started expressing breast milk for Noah. I wanted to breastfeed him very badly and thought it was even more important now because he was sick. Even though he was being fed by a gastric tube, I felt it was the one thing I could do for him. He needed all the extra help I could give him, and it helped me feel that I was participating in some way. It almost felt normal, too. There was nothing normal about the rest of his birth, but it felt normal for me to express my milk for him.

The next day I was released from the hospital. My body quickly recovered from the toxemia and HELLP syndrome. I felt pretty good but knew I had to go home, 350 miles away. The nurses told me that Noah would be fine. He was very stable, and they were even able to wean him off the ventilator a bit. It was horrible saying good-bye to him. I was terrified that I would never see him again. I remember leaving downtown Denver and thinking, "How can I leave my child here all alone?" Of course he was not alone; he had the most wonderful NICU staff I could ever imagine. It still did not feel right. What kind of mother could possibly leave her tiny baby? I knew that it was necessary, but it still did not feel right. I had already made the decision to stay in Denver with Noah, and I had to get my things.

That night sitting in the dark in his room at home in Wyoming, pumping milk for him, all I could do was cry. I was so miserable. I sat looking at his crib and all the clothes that had looked so tiny a week ago but I knew would never fit him. It felt like my heart was breaking. I just wanted it all to go away. I wanted to wake up and be pregnant again, and have a healthy baby. I was in denial. The next morning I put Noah's birth announcement in the paper. It felt like the right thing to do. I needed to let everyone know that I had my son and loved him very much.

I got back to Denver as soon as I could. Noah continued to do very well. When he was about a week old, I finally got to hold him. It was the most amazing moment in my life. I wanted to sit there with him in my arms forever. Again the big blue eyes looked at me as though they knew the world. Somehow I felt that everything was going to be all right. Soon Noah was doing well enough to be moved to the graduate nursery. I was so proud. I finally felt that things were going the way they should. Although Noah was not gaining weight, he was doing wonderfully. I, however, was not. I was beginning to hate everyone who had a "normal" baby. I was also beginning to be very cynical. It seemed to me that no one in the world knew what was really important. Everyone was running around getting mad at people for cutting in front of them at the grocery store or getting slow service. It just wasn't worth it to me. The only thing that mattered was that tiny boy. I would get so angry with people who did not appreciate their healthy children, and even more upset when I heard stories of young girls having babies they did not want. They did not deserve healthy children. All I wanted was a baby, and I got a very sick one; these girls did not want kids but got healthy ones. Looking back, it was very foolish to think that way. I am so thankful now that Noah was born to me and not someone who did not really want a child. Someone who was not totally devoted to a child would have given up on him long ago, and the world would never have known the joy that is Noah.

It was almost Christmas, and Noah had been in the hospital for over a month. I had gone home to attend a Christmas party. In the morning the hospital called saying that Noah was very sick and we should get there as soon as possible. The drive to Denver was pure hell. The nurse who called did not tell us much. I did not even know if my son would be alive when we got there. It seemed that we could not go fast enough. When we finally made it to Denver, we got stuck in a parade. I was so frustrated and scared I could hardly breathe. After what seemed like an eternity, we finally made it to the hospital. When I walked into the hospital room, I thought my heart was going to fall out of my chest. My son was lying there shaking. He could not stop twitching even when I put my hand on him. He looked at me as if asking me to help him, and there was nothing I could do. His wonderful blue eyes had a horrifying glaze. I could not stay in the room. I knew my son was dying. There are no words to describe the feeling of watching your son teeter between life and death. The doctors told us that he was in extreme septic shock. That was all they could tell us at the time, but we should expect the worst.

It was then that I met a wonderful woman named Deb who would get me through a lot of trying times. She had preemie twins. Over the next month we became very close. When she saw my face, she just hugged me and let me cry in her arms. She stood with me as I called my mom and told her that Noah was dying.

I am not entirely sure what happened that night; I think I blacked it out. But, defying all odds, Noah made it through the night. The next day he seemed a bit better. Slowly he did improve. Shortly after that, however, we found out that Noah had suffered a grade IV intraventricular bleed. I was told that a grade V is the worst. This was Noah's second bleed; he had suffered a grade II bleed at birth. The doctors could not tell me what the outcome would be. He did need two spinal taps to reduce the swelling in his brain. They knew from the ultrasound that it would most probably affect his right arm and leg, and he would have some form of cerebral palsy. I can't say that I was surprised. It was scary, though. I grasped at what the neonatologist had told me. He had said that they knew very little about infant brains. He said that kids with grade 1 bleeds can be badly brain damaged and kids with 5's can have very few problems. I clung to that. It was my only light at the end of the tunnel. At that time I promised myself that I would never treat Noah as though he was disabled, no matter what the outcome. I firmly believe that treating a child as though he is disabled gives him a way out, so he does not have to try as hard.

Shortly after Noah's brush with septic shock, I almost had to make the hardest decision of my life. My mother was with me. Noah's father was only able to be with us on weekends, and my mother came whenever she could. A doctor told me that my son's single kidney was failing. There was very little they could do because of his size and other medical problems. The doctor thought we had very little time. My mother had to leave the room. I sat there and let it all sink in, trying to get the courage to call Noah's father. Then a very special priest walked in. Up to now I had been very angry with God. I wondered what I could possibly have done that my innocent baby should be punished like this. I chatted with this wonderful man about my son, and we prayed. For some reason a calm came over me. I am not saying that I was "touched by God," but the priest helped me see that things happen and God has a plan. I felt so much better. My relationship with this priest continued for many months. He always seemed to be there when I needed him, which was so comforting. Over the next few days Noah's kidney took a turn for the better, and so did my attitude. I stopped blaming God and slowly began to realize how lucky I was that Noah had been born to me. I still thank God every day for giving me Noah and allowing him to teach me the things he does.

Noah's condition improved over the next few weeks. We found out that the infection that had caused him to become so ill was a yeast infection in his blood. They are very difficult to treat, much less cure. He would continue on the antibiotics off and on for the next sixteen months to try to cure the yeast infection. We watched him closely for necrotizing entercolitis (NEC). I was sure that he would get it because my poor little guy seemed to get stuck with everything, so I just expected it—but he made it unscathed. He also had an eye exam with no signs of retinopathy of prematurity. The doctors were worried, however, that he was not gaining any weight. By six weeks of age he had not gained any weight. We were very concerned because he could not have his esophagus reattached until he weighed 2.5 kilos, and he was hanging out at about 1.75. I was getting very frustrated. Noah could not come home until he had his esophagus reconnected. It is very hard to feel like a real mother when you leave your child every night for someone else to comfort when he cries.

Christmas was quickly approaching. Noah was once again doing well enough to be moved to the graduate nursery. He was a feeder and a grower again. I told Noah that all I wanted for Christmas was for him to gain weight. Amazingly enough, on Christmas Eve my husband and I went back to the hospital for his night cares. We watched anxiously as he was placed on the scale. He had done it! He had gained half an ounce from the night before. From that day on, Noah consistently gained weight until he was big enough to have his esophagus reconnected.

A very sad thing happened on New Year's Eve. My friend Deb's daughter passed away. She had suffered an infection while her mom was still pregnant. It was more than her little body could handle. The next day she took her little boy home after four months. I could not find the words to tell her how sorry I was. I had seen a few babies die in the NICU but none that I was close to. The worst thing was that Deb had originally been pregnant with triplets. She got to take only one of her babies home. She was an amazingly strong woman who was very grateful for the time she had with her daughter and was so happy to have her son. It was very hard personally to be so close to a baby dying. Children are just not supposed to die before their parents. I thought often of how lucky I was to have my child with me. I realized how vulnerable these children really are—how vulnerable all children are. Every time Noah got very sick, I was terrified that my son would end up like Cassie. It wasn't that I did not already know it was a distinct possibility that my son would die. Outwardly, I was very optimistic that he would survive; inwardly, I was terrified. I thought about him dying every day—almost every moment. But I put on a good front. I would not let my son see the fear in my eyes. I had to be strong so he would be strong.

I quickly learned one of the best lessons about surviving the NICU experience: You cannot spend all your time on the baby. No matter how sick the baby is or how much you feel you need to be there, you *must* take care of yourself. If you get too tired or do not take care of your own health, you will not be able to take care of the baby. Many times I tried to be there all the time, but I soon realized it was too emotionally and physically draining. I was still pumping for Noah and was spending about sixteen hours a day with him, leaving only at shift change. It was too much. No matter how thankful I was that I could be with Noah all that time, I just couldn't be. I found that going shopping for an afternoon, always for baby things, could save my sanity. I also found that pumping was very comforting to me. I got to relax, watch TV, and make phone calls for fifteen or twenty minutes every four hours. It was my little escape. Making time to take care of myself made me better able to take care of my baby and the rest of my family.

Noah had his esophagus surgery on January 15, 1996, and everything went well. They were able to reconnect his esophagus without a hitch. It was very hard to send such a tiny baby to surgery, but I had to trust that God would give the doctors the skill and knowledge to fix my son. After his esophagus surgery, Noah had a very hard time coming off the ventilator. He had developed a condition called tracheomalacia; essentially, his trachea collapsed when he breathed. They decided to do yet another surgery. The doctors tied his aorta to his sternum and stinted his trachea to keep it from collapsing. Noah did very well for a short while, and then his colostomy began prolapsing, or coming out. For about a month Noah went to surgery every weekend. All of these things were due to VACTERLS syndrome, complicated by prematurity. It was very hard—no, hard does not describe the feeling of sending your child to the operating room every weekend. I decided that it helped to look at it this way: He did not know that this was not normal. He did not know that life was not about surgery, being poked, and having machines breathe for him. It was not normal for me, though. I wanted nothing more than to have my son fall asleep in my arms while lying on my bed. The doctors kept promising me that he would be fine after this one last surgery and could then go home. I had to hold on to that. I think I would have gone crazy if I had given up—and I couldn't give up because my son would not give up.

Noah had a very hard time after his series of surgeries. He seemed to get one infection after another and needed to have a blood transfusion every time. Noah ended up having about seventy-five transfusions in his hospital career, and he got blood from a nonfamily member only three times. He got blood from his father, my father, and me. He also got pneumonia. It did not seem to be viral or bacterial, and he was not getting any better. His liver was also beginning to fail. His doctors were afraid that the hole in the septum of his heart, known as an atrial septal defect (ASD), was causing blood clots that could result in lung failure. Then they thought they should check his heart function. He was scheduled for a heart catheterization, which for some reason was scarier to me than regular surgery—for good reason, as it turned out. The catheter brushed Noah's heart wall, and his heart went into an irregular rhythm; they had to shock his heart back into the right rhythm. I was overwhelmed when I realized how close my son came to dying.

Three days later Noah was scheduled for open-heart surgery. He had a hole between the two upper chambers of his heart, and the blood that should have been returning to his heart from his left lung was actually draining into his liver. This meant that only about 25 percent of the blood in his body was circulating, and the rest was flowing back and forth to his liver, heart, and lungs. Ironically, he was given only a 25 percent chance of surviving open-heart surgery but zero chance of surviving longer than a month without it. How was I supposed to send my son into surgery knowing he would probably not survive? How was I supposed to decline surgery when I knew it was his only chance of survival? I had not been surprised to learn he needed open-heart surgery; I had just hoped it could be put off until he was about two years old. But I had not known the full extent of his heart anomalies. The next morning all I could do was cry. Knowing that the next time I saw my son he might be dead was terrifying—so terrifying that I almost could not function. Once again I put my trust in God. I was not in control of the situation. I fell back on what the priest had said: God had a plan. After all, the only thing I had been in control of since my son was born was what I was going to eat.

The next day I watched them wheel my 6-pound son to his eighth surgery, knowing that I might never again see his beautiful blue eyes looking up at me. It was almost more heartache than I could bear. The next six hours were a roller-coaster ride. I was told that Noah might not be able to come off the heart bypass machine. It was very hard on a person's kidneys, and Noah only had one. And there were other questions: Could his body handle the increased blood flow? Could his liver repair itself? Could his heart handle the surgery itself?

We were very lucky that a very special NICU nurse went to surgery with Noah. She came out every hour like clockwork to let us know how he was doing. Finally, she came out and told us everything went well, and his heart started right back up. I could not imagine operating on a heart smaller than an egg, much less manipulating the vessels that came out of it.

After about an hour we were let into the pediatric ICU to see Noah. Children could not go back to the NICU after heart surgery. I had seen my son hooked up to all kinds of machines, but nothing prepared me for this. He was on a ventilator and had at least four IV lines, two pacemaker wires, a gastric tube, a urine catheter, and two chest tubes. He also had a 4-inch piece of tape running down the middle of his chest covering about twenty stitches. He looked like a bad Frankenstein experiment. *But he was alive.* That night his father stayed with him in the hospital. For the next few days we went in shifts so that he was never alone. And he beat the odds. I have always said that if there is an odd out there to be beaten, good or bad, Noah will beat it.

A little over a week later he was extubated. Was this it? Were we on the road to recovery and possibly home? Noah had his first bottle a few days later, at nineteen weeks. But our joy was short-lived. Two days later he had to be reintubated and went back on antibiotics. He also needed new chest tubes. It seemed that the yeast infection was back. This time the concern was that it had seeded in his kidney. Exploratory surgery found only a misshapen kidney. Then Noah began having a reflux problem—finally, a normal preemie thing! Hernia repairs and colostomy revision came next. I was almost at the point where surgery did not bother me anymore. I am almost certain it did not bother Noah. What did bother me was that I was getting to know the anesthesiologist all too well. It is not normal to be able to call your anesthesiologist by his or her first name. I think

I developed a sense of normalcy about it all because it was my life. Noah was now about five months old and was averaging about two surgeries a month. The motherly fear never went away, of course; I think I just learned to cope. And, once again, my baby would not give up, so how could I?

At this point I decided to give up pumping. The pumping room was quite far from the PICU, and it was too stressful. Noah was no longer being fed breast milk because it was too rich for his body to digest. He had been on formula for about two months, but I had continued to pump in the hope that he would be able to breast-feed. It did not look as if that would happen for a while, and we did not know if he would ever be able to tolerate it. I had donated over 1,000 ounces of my milk to a mother's milk bank at the hospital. The thought of helping other babies made me feel good.

Soon doctors discovered that a lymph duct had been accidentally cut in Noah's chest. I was told that it happens in about 5 percent of all open-heart surgery. Once again, my son and the odds! So it was back to the OR. This time Noah was very, very sick when he came back. The lymph that had been draining out of his chest was pooling there. His little tummy was so swollen, it was beginning to crack. I often thought about little Cassie. She had been swollen, too. I wondered if this was God's way of telling me that Noah was going to be with Him now. I knew Noah was in pain; he could not even open his eyes. The doctors told me that his kidney was once again failing. It seemed to be Noah's time to go. I told him in a very tearful and terrifying moment that if it was too much, he could give up. I also told him that he was a strong boy and I knew he could beat it, but I also knew he was tired. I told Noah a lot of things that night—very personal things, things that I was going to tell him when he was older but might not have the chance. In the morning I was going to tell them that Noah had fought long enough. I could not even think about my decision. My brain told me it was the right thing to do, but my heart could not take it. I could not imagine what life would be like without my little boy. I said many prayers that night hoping God's plan somewhat resembled mine. I guess it did. Noah once again beat the odds. When I arrived that morning, Noah's kidney function had dramatically improved. I guess he was not as tired as I thought.

Over the next week or so, Noah got much better. We were then faced with a new dilemma. The doctors felt that Noah would be much more comfortable with a tracheostomy. Noah's tracheomalacia, the collapse of his trachea, had not gotten any better. He could go home with a trach and be relatively normal. It was a very scary thought, but I knew in my heart that whatever the outcome, Noah needed to be more comfortable. He had had a tube down his throat from the moment he was born, more or less. He deserved to be free of that. Surgery number twelve was his trach.

Up until this point I had been able to tell myself that Noah would be just a normal little boy when he got to go home. However, now I knew that nothing would be normal after they cut a hole in his neck. Everyone who looked at him would know he was not normal. I was terrified that people would ask themselves how a mother could do that to a child. I worried that people would think I should have let him die. To be honest, I thought that myself. I often wondered if I should just let him die. Was it fair for me to want a child so badly that I would put him through so many surgeries and so much pain? Every time I looked at that little boy, I knew my answer. It was *no!* He never gave up. He never lost his will to live. Then I would fall back to: God had a plan. God knew that Noah had wonderful things to share with the world. God knew what He was doing. We just had to trust in that.

Noah did seem much more comfortable after his trach. He could finally suck on his pacifier easily. Soon we got his portable home ventilator and Noah was on the move. He could get out of his crib, rock with me, and even sit in a baby swing. I had converted his room in the intensive care ward into a home nursery. He had his own sheets and blankets and posters on the wall, and he even had a six-month birthday party with cupcakes and all his favorite nurses.

Just after his trach, Noah had a neurology consult. The neurologist had the nerve to come into my son's room and tell me that Noah was probably blind and deaf, and would be in a vegetative state all his life. I was furious. I was so mad, I was shaking. At this point Noah had begun seeing life. He had been on morphine for about three months, and they used methadone to get him off. How can any child possibly develop and show any signs of being normal when he is a morphine addict and has been fighting for his life in the hospital for six months? Noah then had eye and hearing tests that came back abnormal. The doctors told me that he could hear and see, but when the signals got to his brain, he could not decipher the signals to know what he was seeing and hearing. I knew that my son could recognize many things.

Despite what the neurologist said, Noah was doing very well. In May and June, Noah got to do some very normal things. He learned to drink from a bottle through a nipple, he went for walks outside, he received occupational and physical therapy every other day, and he even sat at the nurse's desk. It seemed we were on our way home.

Over the next few months Noah was subjected to many more trips to the OR—for little things, though. He had many esophageal dilations, a liver surgery, and a heart catherization—nothing very life threatening. However, Noah began having more problems with his colostomies; they became very fragile and bled a lot. One night I left the hospital at about 10 o'clock, and by the time I returned in the morning, Noah had had four blood transfusions because he had been bleeding so much. His colostomies were fragile because Noah had a form of hepatitis due to being on IV nourishment for so long and from the damage when his heart was not working properly. I was told it would probably repair itself, but in the meantime he needed to have his colostomies removed. The only way to do that was to have an anus made. It went wonderfully, except that he had to have some tissue removed in a later surgery. When Noah was thirty-one weeks old, he rolled from his back to his side. I was probably the proudest mom ever to see her child roll over. About a week later Noah had his colostomies taken down, commonly called a pull-through. I finally got to change a poopy diaper. My son was thirty-two weeks old. It was amazing. He no longer had part of his colon outside his body.

The next three months were very easy for Noah. He was doing relatively well. He had to have a few more surgeries but, again, nothing major. I joked with the surgeons that Noah should have his own OR suite. The three months after that were hell for me. My husband asked for a divorce in July. We had been having some problems, but I thought we could work things out. He told me that the things he wanted out of life were different from mine. I was absolutely devastated. Here we were getting ready to take our son home, and we did not have a home to go to. I did not know how I was going to be a single mom to a disabled child. I could not just take a child like Noah and put him in day care and get a job. I had no idea how I was going to support us. Many marriages that must endure a sick baby do not endure. It was very hard on us being away from each other for so many months. My husband was trying to make some sort of real life, and I was trying to take care of the baby.

In late October, Noah began smiling and making noises. I was so excited. He could react to things normally. I was sure this was a very good sign. I had called my mom a few months before, terrified that Noah would never smile. For some reason the thought of my son never smiling really upset me. It is kind of funny now because all Noah ever does is smile and laugh.

On September 6, after nine months in the hospital, my dream was coming true. We were told that Noah was as well as he would probably ever be, and he was okay to go home. The doctor said there was little more they could do at the hospital. Basically they told me that I should take him home but not expect too much. I was determined to prove them wrong. I knew he would do amazing things if I could just get him home—but that was not so simple. First, I had to find a nursing service that could support twenty-four-hour nursing care, because Noah would be going home with a ventilator, oxygen, food pump, and a central IV line. Next, someone from the nursing service had to meet Noah and get used to all his equipment. Then we had to get all the home supplies. Our doctor in Wyoming wanted Noah in the hospital near home for two days. Finally, it was all set.

On September 23, after forty-five weeks, three days, and thirty-four surgeries (twenty-nine major and five minor), we were on our way home by Learjet. It was very hard leaving the hospital; it was like leaving a security blanket. It was going to be very strange without the full-time staff of doctors and nurses. For some reason, though, I was not scared. I knew my son better than anyone, and I had acquired a lot of medical knowledge. I was ready to have my son home.

Noah was finally home! It was amazing. I could watch him sleep in the middle of the night, snuggle with him on the couch, and take a bath with him. It was the best thing in the world. Noah did very well at home for about a month, then he got an infection in his central IV. We went back to the hospital. We drove to Denver, and Noah was in for a week while they treated his infection. It was very strange returning to the hospital. I had gotten very used to being at home with Noah.

On Noah's first birthday we moved out of his father's house to my hometown where all my family lived; I figured I would need all the help I could get. Noah absolutely blossomed. We quickly got into a routine of being just the two of us. He showed me that he was not blind or deaf. He was still developmentally a newborn, but he was such a joy. It was difficult to go anywhere with Noah; he was on a ventilator full-time, so I had to take it with us wherever we went. It

took about an hour to get ready to go anywhere and was nearly impossible to do alone, but we made it.

Slowly, Noah's trachea began to improve, and he was able to be
off the ventilator for short periods of time—and eventually all day.
His IV line was removed in May. Physical therapists told me his developmental stage was that of a three- or four-month-old. He began
receiving physical therapy twice a week and quickly made progress.

After Noah came home, I met a wonderful man who was very
glad to step in as Noah's father, although Noah's real father sees him
twice a month. Jody was willing to be Noah's full-time father and
support us, allowing me more time with Noah. He is truly a blessing.
I now work part-time, just to keep my sanity. And, yes, I still call the
doctor at every minor twinge and tingle.

Noah has had about five minor surgeries since he has been home,
but he has spent a total of only three weeks in the hospital in the
eighteen months that he has been home. He still has a trach and a
gastric tube. He is no longer on the vent but is on continuous airway
pressure at night. He has a horrible aversion to eating, but I am told
that it is not unusual for a child with his history. He is on very few
medications. He had his central line removed in May 1997. His kidney works great, and so does his liver. Noah had his trach removed
in August 1998 and is doing very well. The two major problems we
have now are diaper rash and bad teeth; his teeth were severely damaged by the high doses of antibiotics he received as an infant.

Noah has developed wonderfully. He is still severely delayed but
shows all signs of eventually catching up. He sits up and tries to
stand. He loves to play drums and peekaboo. All he ever does is
laugh and smile, especially if his papa is being silly. He likes to play
alone and loves to entertain people. He is very good at mimicking
people's actions, and he sees and hears very well. If he cries, something is really wrong. He is a very happy little boy, and he is the joy
of my life. I am a very happy mom.

We still have some very hard times, but it is mostly emotional on my part. I would love to see my little boy run and play with the other kids; however, I know that when he does take that first step, it will mean so much more to me than it would to other people. It is very hard for me to see people who don't realize what a gift their children really are. It is a shame that people take healthy children for granted. It is also very frustrating for me to talk to people who think they understand what we have gone through and what we have yet to go through. I think it is too difficult for most people to comprehend what my son has gone through. I also get very upset when people tell me what an amazing person I am for doing all that I have for my son, how strong I am, and how they would have gone crazy. I tell them that they would have done it, too. I just did what I had to as Noah's mom.

I have a beautiful son and a wonderful man who is willing to share all our ups and downs. I would not trade either for the world. My life is so much richer with Noah in it. He has taught me so many things. He has taught me how really precious life is and what a blessing children are, whether they are healthy or not. He has taught me that I must be patient because things do not always go my way, but the rewards can be so much greater. He has taught me that perfection comes in many different shapes, sizes, and disabilities. I was also taught never to give up. My son and I did not give up despite being told there was no hope, and now we have a wonderful life. I was reading his discharge summary earlier. It said, "The prognosis for Noah is very poor." Once again Noah had beaten the odds. Most of all, Noah has taught me that I am one very, very lucky person.

DUSTIN:
TINY BUT MIGHTY

by Kim Wilson

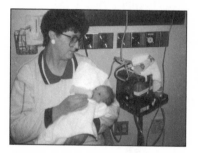

Dustin and his grandma, Susie Lang.

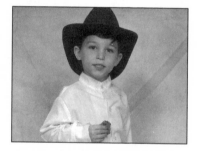

Dustin, five years old.

October 21, 1993, is a day I will never forget. After thirty-two weeks of a pregnancy filled with bed rest, medication, and fetal monitoring, I gave birth in Arizona to my son, Dustin.

I awoke the morning of October 20 to a dampness on the sheet. I had never lost control of my bladder during the pregnancy so I was positive my water broke. I remembered reading somewhere that if a woman's water broke low, she would experience a "gush," and if it broke high, she would experience a slow, infrequent "trickle." Apparently mine broke high.

I called my doctor. He was not surprised to hear my voice; in fact, he had heard it many times during the pregnancy. The baby was due in December, and in June I had gone into labor. Thankfully, we were able to stop the labor with medication consisting of terbutaline and magnesium, along with bed rest.

"I think my water broke," I said to my doctor, and then proceeded to tell him that I was having some slight cramping but nothing severe. He instructed me to get to the hospital immediately. I asked him if I could take a shower.

"No. You can take one when you get here. Just come to the hospital as quickly as possible," he said.

Chuck, my husband at the time (we have since divorced), and I left right away on the twenty-two-mile trip to the hospital. I was already registered, so I didn't bother to call and let them know we were coming.

When we arrived, a gentleman at the desk in the lobby took my name and then called for a nurse to wheel me back. Since I was approximately two months early, they put me in a large labor and delivery room. I was told the room was so large because they would need the space for all the people who would be attending the birth.

"When you're getting close to having the baby, we will call upstairs and a team of neonatal specialists will come down here to assist with the baby after it's born," said the blond nurse. She handed me a gown and requested I change into it.

"If you don't mind, I brought a large shirt. Can I please wear that?" I asked.

"Sure, whatever you're comfortable in. I just need to let you know that in case of an emergency, we may need to cut it off you," she said with a smile. I told her that was fine.

After I changed she started the IVs and hooked me up to an external fetal monitor and a cardiac monitor. Several times they lost the baby's heartbeat on the monitor. They couldn't determine if the monitor was faulty or the baby was truly in distress, so they inserted an internal fetal monitor. To our relief the internal monitor worked much better, although it had to be the worst and most uncomfort-able part of my labor. Soon my doctor arrived and did a test to make sure my water broke. Sure enough, it had.

"Well, within the next twenty-four hours you're gonna have a baby," he said.

I already knew the baby was a boy and that his name would be Dustin. We phoned Chuck's mom, Angie, to tell her I was in labor. She thought we were joking, because two days prior, on October 18, Chuck's sister had given birth to a premature daughter. Chuck's mom would become a first-time grandma twice in one week to two premature babies.

Shortly after I got off the phone, a nurse came in and sat down next to my bed. "Has anyone talked to you about our Neonatal Intensive Care Unit?" she asked, looking at both Chuck and me.

"No," we said in unison, shaking our heads.

"Your baby will be taken there after it's born," she said. "This is a special nursery, and you need to be prepared for it. Your baby will have several tubes and life-sustaining hook-ups. I will take you," she said, pointing to Chuck, "on a tour of our NICU and answer any questions you may have."

Tears filled my eyes. I had never even thought about my baby go-ing to the NICU. Oblivious to everything going on around me, I had just assumed I would have a healthy baby boy who would be in the regular nursery where visitors could stand outside and marvel at him through the glass window. The nurse asked me if I had any ques-tions. I shook my head but wondered how I could have overlooked something so obvious. Chuck left with the nurse for his tour. He re-turned about thirty minutes later with tears in his eyes.

"Those are some pretty tiny babies" was all he could manage to say. Just then the phone rang. It was my mom calling from Iowa for an update.

"Do you and Kim want me to come out right away, or would you prefer if I came out after the baby is home from the hospital?" she asked.

"Come out right away. Kim's going to need you," I heard Chuck say.

Throughout the day my labor continued but did not advance. Around 10 P.M. the decision was made to induce labor. I found this quite ironic because I had spent the past several months doing everything possible to stop labor.

I was on the phone several times that day from the labor and delivery room giving my family in Iowa updates. Everyone was secretly hoping the baby would be born today and share his birthday with his great-grandmother, the same way my brother and great-grandmother shared a birthday, but Dustin had different plans.

At 2:30 A.M. on October 21 the medical team decided it was time to start pushing. The team from upstairs was called down. What seemed like a large room soon became smaller as people started filling in, taking their assigned positions.

"This is gonna be a tiny one," exclaimed the doctor. At 2:56 A.M. Dustin made his entry into the world. He was whisked away without my even seeing him. I tried to capture a look, but all I could see were the backs and masked faces of his caretakers. I kept hearing "Wow" and "I can't believe it" over the humming of equipment. I was too scared to ask what was going on. I just stared at the mass of people surrounding my baby.

Soon a nurse came over and said I had a very healthy 5-pound 7½-ounce, 19-inch baby boy. Chuck and I were stunned, along with everyone else. We were expecting a 2- or 3-pound baby. We were thrilled. And I guess it was a blessing that we didn't know what lay ahead for us.

Chuck had been with Dustin since the delivery. Running back and forth across the delivery room, he kept giving me updates. "He has a lot of black hair," he said, then raced back over to Dustin. A few minutes later he came back to me. "He has all his fingers and toes." Quickly he was gone, racing back over to Dustin.

Thirty minutes after Dustin was born, Chuck and a nurse holding Dustin walked over to me. Smiling, she handed me my precious son. Both his eyes were closed, and I marveled at how cute he was. I gently pulled off the blue cap on his head and ran my fingers through his black hair. I put the cap back on and unwrapped the blue blanket. I wanted to see with my own eyes that he truly had all his fingers and toes. Just as Chuck had said, he did. Dustin started to squirm, and then he opened one eye; not quite sure of his new surroundings, he opened the second eye. I looked down as a pair of navy blue eyes looked back at me. "Hi, handsome," I said, kissing his cheek.

After what seemed like only a few minutes, a nurse came and took Dustin from me, stating that they needed to run more tests on him. Once again God was looking down on Dustin because he was able to go to the regular nursery. This small milestone made it seem as though we were on the right track—but we soon discovered the all-too-common "one step forward, five steps back" way of life of being a preemie parent.

Dustin didn't know how to suck, so the nurses, my mom, Chuck, and I patiently taught him. We played with his cheeks and chin, trying to show him how to develop the sucking mechanism. I wanted to breast-feed, but this turned out not to be an option. Dustin was starting to get accustomed to the small preemie nipples on his bottles and wanted nothing to do with me, so I pumped and he alternately received formula and breast milk. We would get so excited when he took .5 centimeters of milk in a thirty-minute period.

"He may be a small and poky eater, but he burps like a ten-pounder," remarked a nurse.

Late in the afternoon on Friday, October 22, my doctor examined me and said I was doing fine and could go home that evening.

"What about Dustin?" I asked.

"His doctor will be in to talk to you. I'm sure you're aware that he cannot go home with you," my doctor said.

I was aware of this, but the impact of his words made it all the more real. My doctor said I could stay in my room after being discharged until the room was needed, but it might be needed soon because the hospital had no available beds. I decided to vacate the room that evening instead of possibly having to leave in the middle of the night.

Chuck and I waited as long as possible before returning Dustin to the nursery and taking our leave. The time came all too soon. Chuck pushed the bassinet, and I began to carry Dustin to the nursery.

"Ma'am, you must put your baby in the bassinet when you're not in your room or in the nursery," a nurse said to me sternly.

"But you don't understand. I've been discharged, and my baby has to stay here," I sobbed.

"That doesn't matter." Then her voice softened. "Honey, because of our liability laws we can make no exceptions." She continued to explain: "If you were to drop him, we could be held liable, but more important, it's for your protection. We have so many people carrying their own children through here, it would be so easy for someone to steal a baby and not be caught carrying it out. We want to make sure that doesn't happen. We want your baby to go home . . . to you."

What she said made complete sense, but I just didn't want to hear it. I wanted to be an exception to the rule, but I knew that wasn't going to happen.

I kissed Dustin tenderly and told him how much I loved him. Then I gently placed him in the bassinet next to a tiny colorful clown he had received as a gift. Chuck and I made the final trip with Dustin from my hospital room to the nursery.

Even though Dustin's stay in the hospital was brief, I missed him terribly. Few parents can understand how horrible it is to leave your newborn baby at the hospital. The night I returned home, the house seemed incredibly empty. I tried to take comfort in the fact that I was very lucky. I kept reminding myself of my blessing. Dustin would be in the hospital only a short time; some parents had to leave their child in the hospital for several weeks or months.

I found pumping quite an experience. Since I grew up in Iowa, I was around dairy farms quite a bit. I've never felt more like a dairy cow in my life than when I pumped. Because Dustin was a preemie, my milk had a hard time coming in. The lactation nurse asked my doctor to order a special pump for me—one designed to attach to both breasts at the same time. For the first six weeks of Dustin's life this worked well, but after that I naturally dried up. Once again, this broke my heart. Now I couldn't even feed my child breast milk. What I didn't understand was that often the stress of being a preemie parent combined with very little sleep is exhausting to the body, and it is very natural and normal to just "dry up."

Chuck and I were not prepared for Dustin's early arrival. I guess I put quite a bit of trust in the hands of the medical professionals. I assumed that by taking my medication and staying on bed rest, my pregnancy would go close to full term. Wrong. Chuck and I had only the crib and the changing table set up. We had not done much shopping, which resulted in our not having much for the new addition to our family.

Dustin remained in the hospital for a few days, and during that time my mom and I went shopping. We went back to the hospital every three hours for Dustin's feedings. One day at the checkout counter of one store the clerk eyed all the baby stuff we were buying and said, "Someone you know must be expecting." I looked at her and smiled.

"I just had a baby boy," I said proudly.

"Well, where is he?" she asked.

Her statement caught me off guard, and the cold reality of my situation hit me hard! Tears filled my eyes. "He was just born a couple of days ago. He was premature, and he's still in the hospital," I choked out.

Finally, after what seemed like an eternity but was only a few days after he was born, we were able to bring Dustin home. I'll never forget trying to figure out the car seat and how to get such a tiny person fitted in this contraption comfortably. Every car door was open as we tried and finally completed our car seat mission.

We got Dustin home, and everything seemed to be going fine. The doctors put him on a feeding schedule of every three hours, but we were to feed him for only thirty minutes at a time. If we went over the thirty minutes, we were told, he would burn more calories than he was taking in. It broke my heart to purposely stop his feedings. It seemed so cruel, especially since I was his mom, and mothers are supposed to take care of their child's needs.

Chuck and I were absolutely thrilled to have Dustin home. I could finally be a mom like other mothers who bring home a newborn. I found it hard to bond with him while he was in the hospital. I never really had him alone, and I was confined to the nursery's schedule. Dustin and I had a lot of catching up to do.

The first time I bathed him was a memorable experience, one that was caught on videotape. At first I was really nervous about bathing him, but Dustin broke the ice by giving me a shower in a way only little boys can do. "Little boys and their toys" was all I was able to say as I laughed hysterically over this incident.

Because he was so tiny his newborn clothes were huge on him. I laughed so hard while dressing him. I changed his outfit several times a day, not because it was soiled but to take more pictures of him.

When Dustin was thirteen days old, I noticed that he had a slight runny nose. The drainage was clear. I thought it seemed odd that a newborn would catch a cold. He was not running a fever, nor was he fussy. I decided to see if the drainage persisted throughout the day. If so, I would call the doctor. As much as I worried about Dustin, I did not want to be one of those parents who called the doctor for every minor medical issue. This particular day I had some quick errands to run. I left Dustin in the care of my mother, who was still staying with us.

"Now, if he's sleeping, you put him down. I don't want him spoiled when you leave," I told my mother.

"If your mama thinks I'm gonna put you down, she's silly," my mother chirped to Dustin loud enough for me to hear. This was her first grandchild, and I knew she was going to make an excellent grandma. I gave Dustin a kiss, told my mom I would be back in thirty to forty-five minutes, and walked out the door.

When I arrived back home, I found my mom frantic.

"Kim, Dustin quit breathing. He started turning blue. I finally got him to start breathing again," my mom said.

Shortly after I left, Dustin fell asleep, but my mom didn't put him down. I was thankful she didn't listen to me. She noticed he wasn't breathing and that his skin color was turning an ashen blue. As a supervisor in the infant department of a day care center, she knew the proper steps of infant CPR and what to do in case of an emergency. She had just revived him when I returned home. Since Dustin was now breathing, I decided that instead of calling 911 and waiting for an ambulance to arrive, we should take him immediately to the hospital.

We quickly made the twenty-two-mile journey to the hospital, and Dustin was admitted and diagnosed with apnea, bradycardia, and RSV (respiratory syncytial virus). I couldn't help but wonder how many times he had quit breathing and nobody noticed. He stayed in the hospital for almost a week. The tests confirmed that part of his brain and lungs were still a little underdeveloped, but he should outgrow this condition. I will never forget this day because it marked the seven-year anniversary of my grandfather's death. I was angry that Dustin's condition was not discovered when he was born and that he was released and sent home so soon after his birth.

Even though I knew Dustin was a fighter, I also knew we could lose him at any time if God so desired. The thought of Dustin's passing away before being baptized was unsettling to me. After discussing my concerns with Chuck, I called our minister. He agreed to come to the hospital as soon as possible.

When the minister arrived, I explained my hope of having a "real baptism" in a church.

"I can give him what we call a baby's blessing," said our pastor. "That way when he's well enough you can have the baptism you desire."

I appreciated his optimism. I knew deep down if something happened to Dustin before his baptism or blessing, God would not deny his entrance into heaven, but I felt I had to do something or I would be failing Dustin as a parent.

The pastor, my mother, Chuck, and I gathered around Dustin's bed to begin the blessing. Dustin was awake and gazing at us with his big blue eyes.

I looked up as a movement caught my eye. Two of Chuck's coworkers were walking in the door; they had been standing outside the door in the hall for the past few minutes. The woman walked over and gave us a hug, tears in her eyes.

"I'm so sorry. You have our deepest sympathy," she said. Then she looked down at Dustin and back up at us. "What's going on?" she said, shocked.

"We're giving him a baby's blessing," I responded, wondering why she looked so pale.

"He's alive," she said.

"I know," I responded, not knowing what else to say to a comment like that.

"Oh, my gosh, that's great," she said with a laugh. "When we saw the minister standing by Dustin's bed, we thought you were doing some type of last rites ceremony."

Now it all made sense: the tears, words of sympathy, and the shocked look on their faces. We invited them to join us for the blessing, and they did.

Dustin was sent home with an apnea monitor that he set off at least two dozen times a day with real alarms and an additional dozen times a day with false alarms. Nothing will put the fear of God in parents more quickly than being awakened in the middle of the night by the alarm that indicates their child is not breathing or their child's heart has stopped.

When the "real" alarms sounded, we were instructed to call out his name. If that didn't work, we were to blow on his face. If that failed, we were to flick our fingers against his feet. And if that failed, we were instructed to call 911 and start CPR. Several times we had to resort to calling out his name, blowing air on his face, and even flicking his feet.

Dustin continued to gain weight at a slow pace, and other than setting off the apnea monitor, he seemed to be making progress. This continued for the next several months. When Dustin first came home the doctors instructed us not to take him out in public for six weeks. I was adamant about following these instructions and also not letting visitors come to see him. I knew his little body was delicate, and I wanted to reduce the chance of his catching anything. I was shocked when I found out that he had RSV. To this day we still do not know how he contracted it.

When Dustin was nine weeks old, we took him to Iowa to be baptized. During the flight Dustin slept on the tiny tray table that flipped down from the seat in front of me. He even set off his apnea monitor, causing several passengers to panic when they heard that high-pitched alarm.

All of Dustin's relatives on my side of the family were finally able to see him. He was the fifth living generation on both sides of my family. We stayed in Iowa for about a week and then returned to Phoenix.

A few days after we returned to Phoenix, I noticed Dustin was starting to get another runny nose. True to form, he was not fussy and did not run a fever. This time I called the doctor, worrying that maybe Dustin was getting RSV again. The doctor instructed me to keep an eye on him and watch him for a fever. Over the next several days the drainage continued and seemed to be increasing. It was now at the point where he was coughing it up. When I fed him, he started choking on the mucus. I called the doctor back and explained what was happening. He told me not to worry since Dustin was coughing it up, but to continue keeping an eye on him.

Several days passed, and Dustin seemed to get worse. He was vomiting up his formula and copious amounts of mucus. I called the doctor and asked him to see Dustin.

"I would feel much more comfortable if you looked at him," I said. "The mucus is increasing and becoming thicker." I made the appointment for that day.

Dustin's car seat was in the backseat of the car, as directed. On the way to the doctor's office he started coughing and gasping. I pulled off on the side of the road and entered the backseat to look at him. It was clear he was choking and gasping for air. I took him out of his car seat and tried "finger sweeping" mucus out of his mouth. Since he was still breathing, I did not initiate CPR. I completed the nearly impossible task of cleaning mucus out of his mouth. When he seemed to be breathing normally, I put the car seat in the front so I could keep an eye on him as we continued to the doctor's office.

The doctor decided he might have a cold or be allergic to his formula. He changed Dustin to a soy formula and then calculated the amount of cold medicine to give him according to his weight. He told me to call if I had any more questions and had me schedule an appointment for a week later.

The next day Dustin seemed to be the same, not better but not worse. The following day he became sicker. He started choking once again on mucus—this time to the point of turning blue. I called 911, and while waiting for the paramedics to arrive, I frantically tried cleaning mucus out of Dustin's mouth and airway. Since he still had a pulse, I did not start chest compressions but I did breathe through his nose and mouth. His color seemed to improve, but he was still gasping for air. I heard the sirens outside. What I didn't realize was that the fire trucks, ambulance, police, and sheriff were all on their way. I ran outside and handed Dustin to the paramedic, who had barely taken one step out of the ambulance.

The memory of my running out of the house to an ambulance with my barely breathing baby is something I'll never forget. I can vividly remember the lineup of the emergency vehicles in front of the house. The ambulance was first, then the police and sheriff's department, followed by the fire truck. The whole street was lit up with red and blue flashing lights.

We arrived at the hospital via ambulance. Dustin was admitted and for the second time diagnosed with RSV. Upon our arrival to the hospital I called Chuck, who worked at the same hospital. Within minutes we were once again looking at our baby lying in a hospital bed. My heart went out to the little guy, who seemed so small and frail in the pediatric hospital bed. I never left the hospital, not even to go home and shower. I just washed up in the bathroom located in Dustin's room and stayed by him night and day. After almost a week he was able to come home.

We arrived back home with his apnea monitor and a machine to give him breathing treatments every three hours. He recovered from this bout with RSV without any other complications. After this incident we kept a constant eye on him for signs and symptoms of possible RSV. I'm happy to say that Dustin did not contract RSV again. When he was six months old, he was taken off the apnea monitor.

Early in his life I dubbed him my tiny-itty-bitty-little-thing. It got to the point where all I had to do was call him that in a certain tone of voice and his face would light up and he'd give me a deep belly giggle.

Dustin always had a fascination with bubbles. One day around his first birthday I was playing with him, calling him by his pet name, and he looked up at me very seriously and said, "Bubbos." Bubbles!

My child said his first word, and I didn't know whether to laugh or cry. I guess my reaction had something to do with the fact that I always thought his first word would be "Mama." So I laughed and tried to get him to say it again, but all he would do was smile and shake his head.

Dustin is now six years old and attends kindergarten. He is happy, healthy, and a very active little boy. He is behind in his speech and recently tested at a three-year-old level. He goes to speech therapy twice a week and is quickly progressing. Otherwise, he is on target. He was walking at a very early age, ten months (eight months corrected). This totally surprised me.

Teething was a different story. It is safe to say he broke no speed records here. He was one year and two weeks old when I finally saw the beginning of a tooth in his lower gum. At one point I was very concerned about his teeth—or the lack of them—and questioned my dentist. He said this does happen occasionally and if Dustin didn't have any signs of teeth by the time he reached eighteen months, I should bring him in and they would take an X ray to see if any teeth were developing. I'm so thankful we never had to make that appointment. (When Dustin was three years old he was diagnosed with an enamel deficiency. The doctors said this is quite common in children born prematurely.)

Before Dustin was born, I was never able to say that I had one particular hero. Now when I think about heroes, without a doubt mine is Dustin. In his short five years he has fought and won more battles than many people, including myself, do in a lifetime. Regardless of how old or how big Dustin gets, he will always be my hero and my tiny-itty-bitty-little-thing.

MITCHIE'S STORY

by Mitch Shue

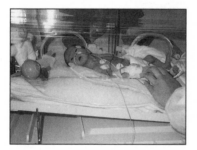

Mitchie, one week old.

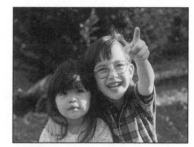

Mitchie, four years old, with his sister, Carly.

It all started on Tuesday, May 10, 1994 (two days after Mother's Day). Oddly enough, we experienced a partial solar eclipse that day. Vickie wasn't feeling too well, but we just wrote it off to her being pregnant and tired. Actually, a few weeks before all this happened, Vickie began to retain water, as many pregnant women do. We were out of town for a baby shower when we first noticed how swollen she was getting. When we returned home, the doctor put Vickie on bed rest for about a week. Vickie's blood pressure was slightly elevated, and, of course, that's not a good thing—especially when you're pregnant. After a follow-up visit, the doctor told Vickie that she required only partial bed rest since her blood pressure seemed to return to normal.

The next Tuesday Vickie just wasn't feeling quite right. I was at work as usual that day, and we spoke over the phone every few hours or so. At about 3:30 P.M. I received a voice mail message from Vickie that I will never forget. I hope never, ever to hear Vickie as upset as she was then. I just knew something was terribly wrong. When I called her back, she told me that she was bleeding and the doctor told her to get to the hospital as soon as possible. I said I would meet her there. Fortunately, our good friend and neighbor Anne was home at the time. Her husband, Bob, with whom I worked, saw me rush out of the office and called Anne. She, who was thirty-four weeks pregnant herself, put their two-year-old daughter in the car and rushed Vickie to the hospital.

I arrived at the hospital just a few minutes after 4 P.M., and Vickie was already in the maternity ward in one of the LDRP (labor, delivery, recovery, postpartum) rooms. We weren't supposed to be there for another eight weeks! One of the nurses quickly put the lead for the fetal monitor in place and located our baby's heartbeat; it was as loud and strong as ever. Needless to say, we were relieved. However, the nurse then told us there was a good chance Vickie was going to have to deliver the baby that day. We looked at each other in disbelief. A few minutes later, based on Vickie's vital signs, blood work, and urinalysis, the doctors decided that both she and the baby were at risk. Vickie had experienced a placental abruption brought on by pregnancy-induced hypertension (PIH), or preeclampsia. An emergency C-section would have to be performed with Vickie under general anesthesia. I kissed Vickie, told her how much I loved her, and then watched them take her into the operating room. Because of the seriousness of the situation, I was not permitted in the operating room but was allowed to look through a narrow glass window in the operating room door. I could see on the faces of the doctors that this was going to be serious.

At 5:42 P.M. on May 10, 1994, our little guy was born, screaming his premature lungs out—a whopping 3 pounds 2.5 ounces (1,430 grams) and 16 inches long. The neonatologist and intensive care nurses were working on him while the doctor continued to work on Vickie. When our son was stable enough, they rushed him to the Neonatal Intensive Care Unit (NICU) just down the hall, pausing briefly to show him to me. I followed our son to the NICU, where I just stared at him in disbelief. He looked so unbelievably little and fragile. They immediately put him on a ventilator to help him breathe. They also connected an EKG/respiratory monitor to him and a pulse oximeter to measure the amount of oxygen in his blood. When they were about to start his first intravenous line, I left the NICU and returned to the hallway outside the operating room to be with Vickie. They were still working on her when I returned. Alarms were going off everywhere, and it was clear to me that something wasn't quite right. It took them what seemed an eternity to bring her out of the anesthesia. I spent the next two hours with her in one of the recovery rooms.

When Vickie came out of the anesthesia, the nurses wheeled her bed to the NICU to see our baby. They took some Polaroid pictures for us, and Vickie was able to hold our baby's hand for the first time. Vickie spent the night in the Critical Care Unit (CCU) instead of the maternity ward because preeclampsia can progress to full-blown eclampsia, resulting in seizures and possible damage to the central nervous system. In addition to medications for pain, the nurses began infusing Vickie with magnesium sulfate to reduce the chance for seizures. Throughout the night the nurses checked Vickie's reflexes by tapping the bottoms of her feet. If her reflexes were too brisk or if her feet "beat" back and forth by themselves after being tapped, it meant there was still a chance for seizures. Vickie's reflexes remained brisk for a couple of days before returning to normal.

I spent the rest of the evening going between the CCU and the NICU. I spent a long time talking with our neonatologist. He explained what was going on with our little boy and that it would probably be a week or so before he was "out of the woods." He explained that it was going to be a rough ride with many ups and downs but that our son should do all right. He was, after all, a pretty good size for being only thirty-two weeks' gestational age. Our little preemie was due on July 6; today was May 10.

After that first night in the CCU, Vickie spent the remainder of her stay in the maternity ward just like mothers who have normal deliveries. Fortunately, Vickie got better and better with each passing day. After nearly three days, we finally named our son Mitchell Alexander, a name we hadn't even considered. Vickie had the final word: "He's a little Mitchie," she said.

Mitchie's first week was pretty rough. Since the respiratory system is one of the last things to develop in a baby, the doctor gave Mitchie a surfactant called Survanta to keep the small air sacs in his lungs expanded. Because of Vickie's complications, Mitchie had a low platelet count that might ultimately have affected how his blood clotted. He was given the steroid Decadron to help develop his respiratory system and to suppress his immune system to give his blood a chance to build up platelets. He was also given Indocin, an aspirin-like drug to help close the patent ductus arteriosus (PDA). PDA is a condition in which the blood vessel that connects the aorta and the pulmonary artery does not close as it should shortly after birth. He was also given triple phototherapy to help him break down his bilirubin because he was jaundiced, as are many babies. For much of the first week Mitchie was blindfolded to protect his eyes from the bililights. The doctor told me that Mitchie would most likely need a blood transfusion before too long since he wasn't able to replenish his blood supply as fast as they were taking it for tests. Since Mitchie was on a ventilator, they would frequently perform blood gas analyses to make sure his system was correctly processing oxygen. Mitchie received all his nutrition intravenously in the form of hyperalimentation and intralipids. The really bad thing about IV sites is that they don't last very long. Mitchie had IVs in his arms, his feet, and his head at one time or another.

We left the hospital on Saturday, May 14, 1994, leaving little

Mitchie behind in the NICU. It was very upsetting to leave him there. Fortunately, we lived just a few minutes away from the hospital and could visit whenever we wanted. We were very thankful for that. We figured that he would get to come home by the first week in July. All he had to do was grow!

Things Go Well . . . for a Little While

The doctors weaned Mitchie off the ventilator toward the end of his first week since he seemed to be breathing on his own quite well. In fact, Mitchie forced the issue by extubating his endotracheal tube. Rather than reintubate him, the doctors put him on continuous positive airway pressure (CPAP) at room air oxygen levels. He received this through a nasal cannula.

Like all newborns, Mitchie lost weight before gaining. He dropped all the way down to 2 pounds 11 ounces before heading in the right direction. Once his system stabilized during his second week, one of Mitchie's neonatologists began introducing breast milk to his diet. We had rented a hospital-grade breast pump so that we could save Vickie's breast milk. The milk was given to him through a nasogastric (NG) tube, a small, thin tube run through his nose and down to his tummy He was given a small amount of breast milk through the NG tube at each feeding. Then after a few hours the nurses would see if he was digesting it by checking his residuals. They did this by drawing back on the NG tube with a syringe. Too much residual was a signal to slow down on his feedings. No residual and sufficient stool were signals to increase his volume.

Mitchie did really well with his feedings and began gaining weight. Toward the end of his second week, Mitchie actually began to breast-feed directly from Vickie! Everyone was pretty amazed that he was able to coordinate his sucking, swallowing, and breathing so well. At this rate he'd be home in maybe three or four weeks. This was when things changed. Toward the end of Mitchie's third week we noticed that his base heart rate seemed to become elevated. He normally hovered around 135–140 beats per minute, but for some reason it was now consistently in the 160–170 range. Every few hours he also began to experience apneas and bradycardias (A's and B's) where he would forget to breathe and his heart rate would drop. This sometimes happens in preemies, but for him it just wasn't normal. Since his hematocrit (percentage of red blood cells) was low and his symptoms could reasonably be explained by this, the doctors decided to transfuse Mitchie. Unfortunately, giving him blood did not improve his condition. The episodes of apnea and bradycardia increased in frequency, and it became increasingly difficult for his nurses to stimulate him to recover. What used to take a little nudge now took resuscitation by "bagging," a process by which the nurses pumped air into him by squeezing a soft bottle placed over his nose and mouth.

On Sunday, May 29, 1994, nineteen days into Mitchie's life, things got much, much worse. The A's and B's increased, his tummy became distended, and he began to have bloody stools. The doctor discontinued Mitchie's feedings and began performing tests to rule possible diagnoses in or out. The good news was that his spinal fluid came back clear, ruling out spinal meningitis. The bad news was that Mitchie showed all the symptoms of a complication known as necrotizing enterocolitis (NEC). We had read about this gastrointestinal complication since it affects premature infants almost exclusively. If left untreated, it could be fatal. Mitchie was getting worse and would have to be transported to a hospital capable of performing surgery on babies as small as he was.

There we were, just barely two weeks after Vickie was discharged and not quite three weeks into Mitchie's life. Vickie was beginning to get around by herself as she recovered from the emergency C-section. We felt more or less recovered from the trauma of a premature delivery and had begun to get our spirits up since Mitchie was doing so well. Our world began crumbling that Sunday. They considered transporting Mitchie by helicopter to the hospital where he was to have surgery, but decided on ground transport instead since traffic seemed to be light. The transport team arrived after 5 P.M. and put Mitchie into a transport isolette (incubator). He was doing so well just two days before that it was hard to grasp the fact that he was so seriously ill. When they were ready to transport him, we were given the opportunity to see him. He was reintubated and barely breathing on his own anymore. He was very still. His eyes were closed. Vickie and I reached into the isolette to touch him, and he opened his eyes. I will never forget his looking up at us. Never.

At about 6 P.M. Mitchie left the hospital. We watched as the ambulance rolled out of the parking lot. When it came to the final stop sign, we saw the lights and heard the sirens go on. We cried for the zillionth time that day.

A Summer Like No Other

After stopping at home to pick up clothes and toothbrushes, we arrived at the hospital well after 7 P.M. We ran into the transport nurse at the elevator, and she told us that Mitchie made the trip without any complications and that he was being stabilized. We were greeted at the door to the NICU by the neonatologist on shift, who talked to us at great length about what was probably in store for little Mitchie. After evaluating his condition and examining his X rays, the surgical team did not feel it was necessary to operate on him immediately. Instead they administered IV fluids and three broad-spectrum antibiotics. We thought then that maybe Mitchie would be okay after all.

We spent the first night in the NICU/PICU parents' waiting room on love seats that were just way too short to sleep on—not that we could sleep anyway. We ended up visiting with Mitchie a few times during the night. The next morning was Memorial Day Monday. Mitchie's X rays did not indicate that his condition was worsening, but clinically he was getting worse. Vickie and I went home to sleep Monday night. Tuesday was absolutely terrible. As we were about to scrub up to see Mitchie, we met Mitchie's surgeon for the first time. He informed us that Mitchie's condition was worsening but that they would continue to evaluate. Later that day he told us that he thought it was time to operate. He had consulted with the attending neonatologist, and they decided surgery would be the best thing. He said the risks of not operating far outweighed those of performing the surgery. A nurse asked us if we would like to contact our clergy. Suddenly the seriousness of the situation really hit us. We started crumbling into even smaller pieces. Vickie and I discussed it for a few minutes, and I began tracking down our pastor to see if he would come to the hospital. We had begun attending our church only a month or so before Mitchie was born. Our pastor arrived sometime around 4 P.M. We held each other while standing around little Mitchie and dedicated his fragile life to the Lord. He went into surgery sometime before 6 P.M. The surgeon said the procedure would take a few hours. That evening a few of our friends showed up at the hospital to be with us. We all prayed for Mitchie and for all the other children in the hospital.

Mitchie came out of surgery around 8:20 P.M. The surgeon came to us in the parents' waiting room to let us know what happened. The surgery had gone well. He told us, however, that he had had to remove a very, very small part of Mitchie's small intestine and more than 75 percent of his large intestine! He also said that they had had a difficult time putting him back together since he was so swollen inside. Mitchie had retention sutures to hold his incision together. The surgeon created an ileostomy as part of the surgical procedure. Mitchie would have to stool into an ostomy bag directly from his small intestine until he was big enough and well enough to have his small intestine reattached to what was left of his large intestine.

Mitchie was in a drug-induced paralysis for several days to prevent him from moving around. He also received medications to control his pain. How Mitchie did over the next ten days was critical to his long-term recovery. Mitchie was pale and bloated from all the fluids they had pumped into him during surgery and would have to pee off all the excess fluids over the next several days as part of his recovery. Since he was paralyzed, he received respiratory support from a ventilator from which he would eventually have to be weaned.

The next several days were tough. All we could do was sit with Mitchie. It was so hard to see him just lying there and not moving—he was attached to so much equipment. Mitchie was on a ventilator for the better part of a week before he could breathe on his own. He came off the ventilator on Monday, June 6. Just when we thought he was recovering, the nurses informed us that Mitchie's right lung had collapsed. For the next week or so they had to perform physical therapy on his little chest to stimulate his right upper lobe. They used the equivalent of an electric toothbrush with a pad on it to vibrate Mitchie's chest. The key to Mitchie's recovery was to keep him free from infection for the next several weeks, no average task. It was difficult to handle Mitchie with all his IVs, the bag, and all the alarms. It was unnerving, but we began doing a lot of the well-baby tasks such as bathing and diapering him. All we had to do now was wait for Mitchie to get bigger and stronger so that the surgeons could reconnect his small intestine to what remained of his large intestine.

Over the next several weeks we developed relationships with a great many doctors, nurses, workers, and parents like us. There were so many children and so many stories. Some had wonderfully happy endings; some were devastating. Since it was a teaching hospital, we saw a new rotation of interns and residents every month. This drove us crazy. We grilled all the new doctors, and I think we gained a reputation for being "hypervigilant," as one of the doctors noted in Mitchie's chart. Soon after they realized that we read all of Mitchie's chart every day, the doctors must have requested that his long chart be removed from his room. We then had access only to Mitchie's daily flow sheet. We became quite the little doctors ourselves. In fact, one doctor asked me if I was in the medical field. We spent so much time in the NICU that we even started watching out for other children.

Countdown to a New Beginning

The surgery to reconnect what was left of Mitchie's large intestine (reanastomosis) was scheduled for Monday, July 11 (my father's birthday). We had been waiting for this day for so long. Once he was reconnected, it would only be a matter of maybe three or four weeks before he could go home—barring any complications, that is.

We arrived before 8 A.M. on Monday so that we could see Mitchie before he went into surgery. When we arrived, we noticed that his heart rate was around 100 beats per minute, pretty low for a baby his size. When the nurse took Mitchie's vital signs right before he went to surgery, as a matter of procedure, we discovered that he was hypothermic—his body temperature had dropped to around 96 degrees Fahrenheit! This was not a good sign since hypothermia, like fever, indicates the possibility of serious infection. The attending physician was notified and came into Mitchie's room with an entourage of residents. A complete septic workup was ordered to rule out infection. Mitchie was immediately put on antibiotic therapy and, as you might have guessed, the surgeon told us that surgery would have to be delayed until Mitchie's condition improved. We were devastated; it was another major setback. Fortunately, surgery was delayed only a week; his cultures came back negative, and after a day under the warmer, he seemed to be just fine.

Mitchie went into surgery on Monday, July 18. It would take a couple of hours to complete the reconnection. A few hours passed, and we didn't hear anything. More time passed with no word. We started to get pretty tense, so I left the surgical waiting room and started walking the halls. I turned the corner to see the surgeon at the other end of the hall walking toward me with his lunch! Isn't he supposed to be operating on Mitchie? It turned out that he had looked for us in the NICU waiting room and not the *surgical* waiting room. He told us the good news: The operation was a complete success, and Mitchie would be returning to the NICU breathing on his own with no help from a ventilator. He would receive his nutrition intravenously while he healed. Now we just had to wait for him to poop. That would indicate that everything was working correctly again, but it might take a week or so. I received a call at work three days later: "Your son pooped!" It sounds funny, but we were ecstatic. Mitchie resumed feeding on Sunday, July 24. He received just a tiny amount every few hours. Every day he received a little more, and on Thursday, July 28, he started getting dried banana flakes mixed with breast milk! He loved it, and he progressed remarkably well. By Friday, August 5, he was consuming about 3 ounces every three hours.

We expected Mitchie to be discharged sometime around mid-August, but we received a call from the hospital on Friday morning, August 5: "You can take your son home today!" they said. We were totally in shock. Vickie and I decided that she would spend Friday night in the hospital with Mitchie, and then we would take him home on Saturday, August 6. Friday night was kind of scary. Vickie and Mitchie spent the night together alone for the first time ever. Vickie was to do everything a normal mom would do. Only Vickie could stay in the parents' room, so I went home to prepare for Mitchie's homecoming.

Homecoming

We put Mitchie in his car seat and said our good-byes to the nurses on shift Saturday morning. Unfortunately, some of the nurses we had become closest to weren't there to see Mitchie go home. It was weird to leave after being there for so long. It was surreal. There were many days when we thought he'd never make it.

Eighty-nine days after he was born and weighing a whopping 6 pounds, Mitchie finally came home. During those eighty-nine days Mitchie had more than sixty nurses and twenty or so doctors care for him. He had survived two major surgeries, had over twenty different procedures performed on him, and consumed over thirty different medications. His medical bills totaled nearly $300,000.

We turned onto our street at around 11:30 A.M. and arrived at our house to a wonderful crowd of our friends and neighbors. I had hung a big banner across the front of our house. It simply said MITCHIE IS HOME!!! And so began Mitchie's precious life. To God be the glory.

Today, Mitchie is just a bundle of joy! You'd never know that he had such a rough start. He does have some food allergies that we have to deal with, but those are minor compared to what Mitchie went through to live. On another happy note, we were blessed with our second child, Carly, on April 19, 1996. Guess what? A normal pregnancy and a normal delivery!

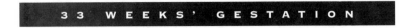

FIGHT FOR LIFE:
BRAYDEN'S STORY

by Trish Brown

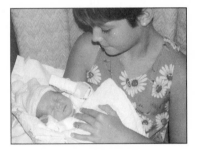

Brayden, seven days old, with his sister,
Laurel.

Brayden, fourteen months old.

During and after my first pregnancy in 1987, I received RhoGAM to
treat my Rh incompatibility. When my daughter was born, she
tested positive for D and C antibodies. My pediatrician was concerned and monitored her for an additional two days before dis-
charging her. After she was released, she never had any problems.
The pediatrician warned me that because I was Rh negative, any future pregnancies might be difficult and have an uncertain outcome.
At that time my husband and I had no plans for any more children,
so this wasn't an issue.

After a time I changed my OB-GYN and discussed this issue with
my new doctor. He said the levels were considered normal as a

reaction to the RhoGAM given during the pregnancy, so we certainly were able to have more children if we decided. My husband and I still weren't interested in the idea. We liked the thought of being able to give everything to our daughter: time, attention, and money.

When my daughter turned eight, my hormones began talking to me. After much thought I was sure I wanted another baby, so I began to broach the idea to my husband. It took him about six months to agree. I had a Norplant that had another year left, so we decided to wait until its removal and then get pregnant. After the removal appointment had been scheduled, I also made a pre-pregnancy appointment. My doctor is very conservative and agreed with me that, considering the past confusion, an antibody screen was in order for peace of mind. Imagine my horror when the "for peace of mind" test came back with high levels before I ever conceived! My doctor couldn't get rid of me fast enough! I was referred to a perinatologist at a large hospital about sixty miles from my home. This turned out to be a godsend. I knew I had a good doctor when my perinatologist spent over an hour with me in consultation. He was not put off by my lengthy list of questions. He pointed out that we had a 50 percent chance of having no problems because the baby might be Rh negative, as I am. However, he was not shy about admitting the potential problems and outlined them thoroughly. He was encouraging in his obvious competence and warm manner.

We decided to begin by repeating my antibody screen just in case. Of course it was still high. We cannot determine how I became sensitized. I have never had a miscarriage that I am aware of and did receive RhoGAM as prescribed at the time. It was theorized that maybe I needed a higher dose than was given. My husband was tested to determine whether he is heterozygous (carrying both positive and negative genes, meaning the baby could be either positive or negative) or homozygous (able to give only negative genes). Thankfully, he was heterozygous, meaning we at least had a chance for a normal pregnancy. My perinatologist gave us the go-ahead to try to conceive, reminding me of the possible risks and telling me to prepare myself just in case.

In early March I was officially pregnant. We were delighted and spent about six weeks in ignorant bliss. I had very mild morning sickness with my first pregnancy, so I was a bit taken aback by the way I felt with this child. It was obviously a different ball game. Thankfully, the nausea subsided by the third month. I continued my aerobics and Nautilus four or five times a week.

The very first antibody titer came back borderline. When repeated a month later, an amniocentesis was already necessary to be clearer on the baby's condition. At this point I crashed, just as my dear perinatologist had warned me I would. I had been so sure we would beat the odds, but we hadn't. All the information I had gathered and was so sure I wouldn't need now became vital.

During all this time I was afraid to jinx anything. I didn't buy any baby items at all and bought only regular clothes in larger sizes, no maternity items. For whatever reason my weight gain was minimal, only eight pounds in all, so most people were unaware I was expecting. My daughter was excited and did most of the informing for us.

Each week was an accomplishment. Our goal was thirty-four to thirty-six weeks. At twenty-four weeks the first of four intrauterine transfusions was necessary. This is an amazing procedure. As during an amnio ultrasound, guidance is used. The needle is placed in the umbilical vein and the baby's hematocrit is sampled. After computation, donor blood is given to raise the baby's hematocrit to an acceptable level. You can watch the baby become more active as the blood is given.

My perinatologist is a no-nonsense kind of guy, and he prefers to do the procedure with an epidural for Mom. I am a control freak and wasn't keen on the idea. We compromised and agreed to do the first one with an epidural and talk about it before the next one. The best description I have after much thought is that at worst it is like a bad IV insertion. It is a bit odd when the uterus is punctured because it involuntarily spasms, but otherwise it's no big deal. For me the procedure itself was amazing. It is fairly unusual in this day of RhoGAM, so we always had an apt audience of various staff people, and on one occasion there was a roomful of interns. As far as I was concerned the worst part was the bed-bound monitoring for six hours afterward to be sure contractions didn't begin.

I made the sixty-mile trip at least biweekly but often several times a week. As thirty weeks neared, the fact that I was going to have a premature baby began to frighten me. I searched everywhere for printed material but found little. What I did find scared me to death, even for a thirty-four-weeker. A consultation with a neonatologist was arranged, and it reassured me only slightly. It is obvious that the variables are great and there are no absolutes in the preemie world. I also decided at this point that I needed to know the baby's sex. We had not wanted to know previously because with so much technology involved I wanted something to be the old-fashioned way. Since white males statistically don't do as well, we needed to know what we were in for. Of course it was a boy, adding to my tension.

At thirty-two weeks my perinatologist decided to take his first vacation in three years. At my regular appointment his new associate determined the baby wasn't doing well and needed an "unscheduled" transfusion. This was the baby's fourth transfusion. We also tested his lungs to see if they were mature. They weren't. The associate's technique was much different from what I was used to. Perhaps the umbilical cord was friable from so much cumulative manipulation, or maybe it was the force I felt that was used. Whatever the reason, there was bleeding into the uterus. It was stopped relatively quickly, but contractions began and didn't stop. The standby terbutaline was tried with little effect. I spent two days on increasing amounts of magnesium sulfate. It was unanimously decided we were as far as we were going to get this pregnancy to go. We scheduled an induction for three days later, allowing time for lung maturation and my perinatologist to return from his vacation.

About midnight the baby began to show distress, so a cesarean was done. My husband had gone home for the night and didn't make it back in time. A couple of the nurses on duty had been with me during the transfusions and understood my control issues, so they set up a mirror to allow me to see the procedure. These nurses also stayed with me in the operating suite. As they opened the uterus, the amniotic fluid was very bloody. I will always remember the anesthesiologist saying, "Oh, my God!" My son's Apgar scores were 9-9, and he was crying! He wasn't shown to me, but was whisked off to the NICU. I knew, though, that he would ultimately be okay.

As luck would have it, the neonatologist who had consulted with me was on duty that night and handled my son's admittance. He talked to us while I was in recovery. He said that the baby was in the best possible condition, and the cord around his neck caused the distress. We were looking at two weeks in the hospital, it was hoped. The baby was on room air only, and required another transfusion because of the Rh incompatibility.

The first three days were a bit scary. We had several false alarms about abnormal test values, ultimately due to either the magnesium I had been given or the Rh process. Brayden spent several days under bililights because his hemolytic process was even more stressed by the abnormal breakdown. On his second day he needed a ventilator because he was tired out. He removed the tube himself the third day and only needed CPAP for a day after that.

When Brayden was three days old, I was allowed to hold him for the first time. His angel nurse for the night was oh-so-tolerant of my spending the wee hours at his bedside. The lab reports were coming back more encouraging, the apneas were subsiding, and his platelets were stabilizing as the magnesium sulfate left his system. After reading and translating the latest report for me and then doing his care, his nurse pulled the curtains and laid him on my chest. It seems trite to say this, as I have heard so many preemie moms repeat it, but there was no one and nothing else but me and him. To say it was glorious would not be strong enough. I cried and laughed and thanked God. It lasted probably twenty minutes but seemed at once to be a split second and forever. I went back to my room and tearfully called my husband, who was home with our daughter.

While in the hospital I spent quite a bit of time with Brayden. I wasn't able to sleep much, so I would walk down to the NICU and stay there until shift change. I was blessed with a lack of pain, never even requiring a Tylenol. On my second day post-surgery I requested early discharge so I could go home and rest. Once home I was confronted with another problem—being away from my son.

At least once a day, and sometimes twice, I would drive the sixty miles to see my baby. I was calling the NICU several times each shift and pumping every three hours. My daughter never knew who might pick her up from school or dance. On the fourth day I called the NICU after I got home late only to find Brayden wasn't there! He had been moved to Special Care. In rapid succession the IVs were removed, the feeds were fully oral, and talk turned to his going home.

On my husband's fortieth birthday Brayden was eleven days old and discharged from the hospital. When I asked the neonatologist about the Respigam series, a medication to prevent RSV, she said not to worry, he wasn't a candidate. Take him home and enjoy him! During our trip home Brayden was an angel even through rush-hour traffic. He was eager to nurse when we got home. Snug in my rocker with my cat beside me and my baby peacefully nursing, I thought we were finally out of the woods. Unfortunately, we would come much closer to losing him once he was home and out of the hospital.

The pediatrician who cared for my daughter did not want to see Brayden until he was home a month. At Brayden's first checkup with her, he was drastically anemic and required the first of many transfusions. This treatment was performed at our local hospital and was horrible for both my son and myself. We asked to be referred to a hematologist. Our request was granted, and we were referred to a doctor who happened to be in Orlando where Brayden was born. The Rh antibodies are supposed to leave the baby's system within eight to twelve weeks. As my son reached twelve weeks he was still becoming anemic. I received a call after hours from the hematologist (also an oncologist) informing me that a pathologist thought the most recent tests showed leukemic cells. A bone marrow biopsy was needed from my three-month-old son. After a sleepy night and an emergency procedure, it turned out to have been a bad reading. All that for nothing!

At least once a week and sometimes as many as four times, I drove my baby over sixty miles to the hospital, held him down so the nurses could put a line into his scalp, and sat waiting for the lab results to find out if another transfusion was necessary. Finally at five and a half months the antibodies had cleared Brayden's system. He is now maintaining his blood counts on his own, and the hematologists have declared him cured.

Today Brayden is 18 pounds at eight months old. He is developmentally on track for his chronological age. To my great surprise he is an exceptionally happy baby. I would think children who have suffered so much would be wary of strangers or have low-key personalities. Not Brayden. He is a happy boy, goes to work with me daily in my pet shop, and smiles at everyone. At school where I do a lot of volunteer work, he happily goes from one person to the next. He has not been sick at all.

I'm afraid I have not fared as well as the baby. I am a member of several Internet lists on prematurity. What I forced my child to endure horrifies me more as time passes, rather than less. I absolutely adored my perinatologist and still do. I believed him when he said that things would be okay, and they are. It is probably a blessing that I was as ignorant of prematurity and its problems as I was. Brayden is such a joy and might never have been born had I known what he would have to go through. I would love another child. For someone who was once sure one was enough, I greet every milestone with both joy and sadness. I am sorry to see my baby grow up. I feel as if I was cheated out of most of his infancy because I was so involved with his day-to-day crises. I hope putting my story into words will help someone else who encounters this fairly rare problem.

AIDAN'S ARRIVAL

by Janice L. Armstrong

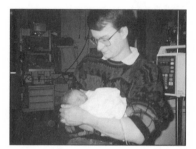

Aidan, one day old, with his dad.

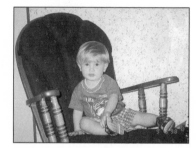

Aidan, twenty months old.

It was with a combination of tears and laughter that I greeted the news I already secretly knew in my heart: I was pregnant. The life growing within me would be my first beloved child. I was just five weeks pregnant when I found out the joyous news, and I knew the remaining thirty-five weeks of my pregnancy would be a wondrous and magical time.

I never entertained the thought I would have a premature child. I did expect some problems. I was overweight and there is a history of diabetes in my family, but I never expected the problems would begin so soon. One day early in my pregnancy my husband and I were watching TV. I had my legs draped across his lap and his arms rested on my legs, our usual position. It felt as if he was digging his elbow into my leg, so I asked him to move. When I looked, his elbow wasn't resting on me at all. He lifted his arm, and we saw a dent in my shin about the size of a tennis ball that wasn't going away. I was eight weeks pregnant. Edema like this cannot be normal this early in pregnancy.

I had to change my general practitioner with this pregnancy because my regular doctor no longer delivered babies. I wasn't scheduled to see the new one until I was twelve weeks pregnant, so I didn't know whom to call. I ended up meeting my new doctor early. He checked out my pitting edema and took my blood pressure, which was high. I was ordered to rest twice a day for one hour each time with my feet up, cut sodium out of my diet, and come back in two weeks. At ten weeks I was still swollen, and my blood pressure was still elevated. I was told that for the rest of my pregnancy I needed to watch my diet and rest.

The weeks passed very slowly, and soon the edema became normal to me. I passed the first trimester, foolishly bragging I had no real morning sickness. I only felt a bit queasy if I neglected to eat regularly. Week fifteen brought the morning sickness! I threw up at least once a day for the next seven weeks. My blood pressure stayed the same, pretty much high but manageable. Despite the discomforts I loved being pregnant—especially after the heartbeat was audible with the Doppler.

During my appointment at eighteen weeks we discussed doing my one-hour blood glucose test early. I was having symptoms of diabetes (although this was hard to differentiate from normal pregnancy symptoms), such as excessive thirst and urination, and feeling dreadful after eating some foods. Because of my history I had already cut out sweets. Just as I knew I was pregnant, I knew I already had gestational diabetes. I failed the one-hour test and took the three-hour test. I knew when I was almost passing out at the lab that I was really not doing too well processing the glucose.

The next morning the doctor's office phoned and said they needed to see me. In the meantime I had read everything I could find online about gestational diabetes. At the doctor's office I was

told I had failed all four values of the test and would need to be under the care of an obstetrician because my pregnancy was now considered "high risk."

I was on a diabetic diet for only three days before it was decided I
needed insulin. I was now seeing on a regular basis a GP, an OB, the
diabetes clinic, and an endocrinologist. I had on average two or
three medical appointments per week from twenty weeks in my
pregnancy on. My OB had me carry my chart with me in case anything went wrong; this way my whole medical team knew what the
others were doing. They all joked that being pregnant was my full-
time job.

I quickly learned how to cope with being a gestational diabetic
and still enjoy being pregnant. I was testing my blood glucose levels
seven times a day at first (it went down to four times per day) and
was injecting insulin four times per day. My insulin requirements
kept increasing despite my strict adherence to the diabetic diet. My
OB was getting "twitchy," as I liked to call it, for he was sure I was
going to have placental problems due to the enormous amounts of
insulin I needed. At each appointment he went through the protocol I was to follow if my BGLs (blood glucose levels) bottomed out
and wouldn't come back up. I thought he was being overcautious
since the endocrinologist didn't think I would have problems. I still
never really considered I could have a premature baby.

Around twenty-eight weeks my blood pressure was on the rise a
bit at each appointment. There were times when I had to lie in the
exam room and rest before they would retake it and allow me to go
home. I was asked about headaches and seeing stars and all those
symptoms that go along with high blood pressure. As Christmas
came my doctor gave me his schedule of on-call days and told me to
go to the Labor and Delivery unit if I had any trouble.

At thirty-two weeks, on New Year's Day, my husband and I were
watching a video. I noticed my Braxton-Hicks (false labor) contrac-

tions were getting rather persistent. I asked my husband to fetch me a large glass of water, knowing this could slow them down, and timed them as we watched the movie. He had no idea what I was doing. In twenty minutes I had four contractions, one every five minutes. I told my husband what was happening. We located my pregnancy books and looked up preterm labor. According to *What to Expect When You're Expecting* I was *not* having contractions. We kept timing and they kept coming every five minutes, but only in my tummy. I decided to take a shower to try to stop them. I went down the hall toward the bathroom and experienced my first taste of what labor would be like. I needed to hold on to the wall during this one. I told my husband to phone Labor and Delivery to see what they said. I was told to come down.

It was 11 P.M. when we got to L&D. The nurse assigned to assess me laid her hand on my belly and commented I seemed pretty relaxed. I told her the contractions had stopped on the way over. She looked at me as though I were a crazy first-time mom who had no idea what her body had been doing, and hooked me up to the monitor. She told me she doubted I had been in labor, but they would continue to monitor me until the OB on call could check me— which was in about an hour. As soon as he inserted his fingers, he said, "Wow, you *have* been contracting all day. By my guess your cervix is very low and fully effaced." He added, "Oh, we have some bloody show as well." The nurse did have the grace to look abashed. He admitted me to the hospital and told me if the contractions came back during the night and couldn't be stopped, I was to be airlifted to Vancouver (a four-hour drive) on the first flight that managed to get out (the weather was very bad).

Now it really sunk in that I might be having a baby prematurely, and it might not all be as okay as I had thought. A friend I had met online who was due a few days before had delivered her son on Christmas Day at thirty-two weeks. He weighed 2,090 grams. I think his safe arrival had colored my perspective a bit about preemies—until they talked about taking me to a different hospital. Then I knew things could be serious even at thirty-two weeks.

The contractions stayed away due to the IV they gave me, and two days later (Friday) I was allowed to go home. The OB who admitted me released me because I had an appointment to see my GP on Monday. Now my blood pressure was more of a problem than my gestational diabetes. My doctor wanted to admit me to the hospital on a couple of occasions, but he always let me stay out when I promised to rest at home. During one appointment my doctor was on call at the hospital. His nurse had taken my blood pressure and made me lie down, then called him. He really wanted me to be hospitalized, but I did not want to go. He said if I agreed to go to the hospital for some blood work and it was normal, I could go home. I didn't realize at the time he was looking for HELLP syndrome. The blood work was normal, and I was allowed to go home. At thirty-three weeks he checked me and found I was 2 centimeters dilated. I never asked him why he had decided to check me. I suspect now that during the exam he felt me contracting.

Two days later I knew my blood pressure was climbing because I was starting to see the stars he was always asking me about. I went to my appointment with a heavy heart. I didn't know if I could talk him into keeping me out of the hospital, but my friend had planned a baby shower for me that Sunday. With strict orders to stay in bed except for three hours on Sunday for my shower, he let me go home, to return on Monday.

Monday I knew it was time to be admitted. So sure was I that I took my hospital bag in the car with me to my appointment. I knew I could sweet-talk him no longer! I was admitted to the hospital for pregnancy-induced high blood pressure that afternoon. I had twice-daily nonstress tests and hoped my blood pressure would go down. I hate the hospital and made my doctor promise that I would not be there until delivery but only until my blood pressure showed some improvement. Tuesday evening my pressure was indeed going down, and he said if it continued, I could go home Thursday. I was so happy!

Wednesday I had to waddle around my baby's head. I had been carrying low, but now he was fully engaged. My contractions were still pretty regular, but no one was terribly concerned about that. As usual I was monitoring and administering my own insulin requirements. After lunch I got the telltale tingling around my lips that signaled a low blood glucose level. I decided to test. Yes, it was very low, the lowest I had ever had. My mom was there, and I asked her to get me a chocolate bar and some juice. I was not recovering as normal. Dinner arrived, and I burst into tears. I was crying hysterically (a side effect of a low-blood-sugar attack). My nurse was at dinner, and her replacement could not figure out how to help me. Finally she got my nurse from her break, and I managed to convey that I didn't know how much insulin to administer. She phoned my endocrinologist at home, and I was taken to the nurse's station to talk to him myself. "Give yourself half your usual dose and have the nurses phone me your after dinner reading" (I test one hour after eating). After dinner my numbers were still too low. Neither the nurse nor I knew at that time that my doctors had spoken about my attack. The nurse came back around 9 P.M. and said that my doctor wanted me in the case room overnight for continuous monitoring.

I was moved around midnight, but instead of being wheeled into the case room, I was taken to labor room 3. At this point I knew I was to be a mom to a preemie. When my new nurse came to check on me, I asked her if the doctor was going to induce me in the morning. She thought that was quite likely. At 1:30 A.M. I phoned my husband to come after he had finished work (we owned a custodial company, and he worked nights). I was very surprised to see him at 4:15 A.M. (he must have flown).

At 7 A.M. a nurse told me I was to be induced that morning. I got a few things from my room, had a shower, and waited. I really was not all that nervous. I thought my doctor was wonderful, and I trusted him. At 8 A.M. my doctor came into my room. I promptly reminded him that my blood pressure was down, and he had said I could go home Thursday if it was. He laughed and told me he knew I was going to give him a hard time about that. I asked him in all seriousness if my baby would be all right being born at thirty-five weeks. He reassured me that the baby would be fine. I now know that a doctor's version and a mother's version of "fine" can be quite different.

At 8:05 A.M. my initiation began with the breaking of my water. Wow, is that ever a strange feeling! The fluid was much warmer than I had expected. I could feel it gush with the contractions, which were still quite numerous all on their own. I was put on an oxytocin drip to get the contractions to work harder. An internal monitor was attached to the baby as well. My contractions were every two minutes but still bearable. At 11 A.M. I was allowed to use the bathroom and walk for half an hour. I wandered over and saw my roommates, for I felt fine! For some reason my teeth began to chatter, and my body shook as if I was cold. Again at 1 P.M. I was allowed to use the bathroom and walk. The contractions were stronger, but I could handle it. Halfway through my walk I hit true labor and wasn't so fine anymore!

I was not sure how I could get back to my room. The walk seemed daunting. I got about 30 feet before a contraction necessitated my holding on to the walls. I made it to my room but could not climb back into the bed. I leaned over it, and my husband began pressing on my lower back. The nurse came in and said, "Oh, there is a sight I like to see. That walk must have done some good." By now my teeth were chattering uncontrollably, and my whole body was shaking. We don't know what caused this, but I shook until I gave birth. The nurse thought I was seizing at one point because I was shaking so bad. She began talking about pain medication, but I said I was fine.

My GP came in around this time and decided to check me. Four centimeters. I was devastated because I had started this at 2 centimeters. I was at about my limit for pain, and it was going to be hours more! My contractions were every ninety seconds and lasted sixty seconds. I agreed to an epidural. Had I known my hard labor was going to be only three and a half hours, I could have made it without the epidural, but hindsight is 20/20.

The epidural lasted only forty-five minutes, and I was feeling pain again. At 5 P.M. I was commenting on the pain way down low. I had a new nurse who was not as experienced. When she finally checked me, at around 5:25 P.M., I was "nine with a lip"! She wanted me to push, but I wanted to wait for one of my doctors. At 5:30 P.M. my OB poked his head in as he was donning his scrubs, and my GP was right behind him. After thanking me for waiting until office hours had finished (!), he told me to push. Three pushes later Aidan Stuart was born, at 5:35 P.M. I looked at him and said, "It's a boy." I lay back until I heard my doctor say, "Maybe it got the knot during delivery." I sat up and looked, and there in the middle of my son's cord was a very tight knot. My doctor said it was a true knot. We are very lucky to have had Aidan at all.

I was allowed to hold him briefly before he was taken to the NICU. My delivery was so fast that the pediatrician missed it, so they wanted Aidan to be evaluated right away. His Apgar scores were 8 and 9, and he was 2,080 grams (4 pounds 9 ounces).

After I had my shower, we waited very impatiently for my paperwork to be done so I could be moved back to the ward. Once there we quickly settled in, then headed to the nursery to see our son. When I got there, I pushed my IV pole over to him and stared at him on the table as though I was in a dream. This couldn't be real. Could this really be my child, the one I knew so well, the one who should still be in my warm belly? He had monitors hooked up to him and a glucose IV inserted, but he was breathing on his own. I took this all in. I was in a fog, silent tears streamed down my face, and I gripped my husband's hand. My joy was mixed with sorrow and fear. My beloved son, Aidan, was here.

Around 9:30 P.M. Aidan was moved to an isolette, and I was allowed to hold him. I was settled in a rocking chair, and he was brought to me. A nurse pulled his IV pole and maneuvered it around mine. I remember wishing that my first time holding him wasn't so awkward, with us both hooked up to IVs. He felt so warm and so right in my arms. As I held him and studied every inch, a nurse told us he would likely be there until his due date and that he was healthy but needed to learn to wake up, eat, and gain some weight. For some odd reason she also told us girl preemies did better than boys. I have no idea why she chose to share that with us. It made us feel horrible, and in fact I was a bit mad. I whispered to Aidan that "we would show her." Reluctantly, I asked my husband if he wanted to hold him, too. When I saw them together, I knew we would get through this. Too soon we were told he needed to go back in his isolette. We stayed and watched him sleep for a long time. I am not sure of the time, but it was late when we left—me to my room and my poor husband to an empty house.

At 5:30 A.M. (twelve hours after his birth) I returned to the nursery. I was struggling to hold Aidan again, doing the IV shuffle by myself, when a nurse said she was going to see if my IV could come out. Even though it was supposed to stay in a few hours more, they took it out. I was then allowed to try to nurse. Aidan took the nipple in his mouth and promptly fell asleep. I nuzzled him so he would be familiar with the smell of my breasts. Later that day I asked if I could begin pumping my breasts to stimulate milk production. I tried nursing Aidan a few times during the day; though we were never very successful, I wanted to persist. Around dinnertime his IV came out. We were told he hadn't needed it because his blood glucose levels turned out to be normal. Of course now they wanted to begin feeding him. He had to start with formula because I still had no milk. As my colostrum came in, they added the few drops I could pump to his bottles. We were still feeling overwhelmed but coping.

The morning of the third day in the NICU I went into the nursery to see Aidan's "twin," as they called the other preemie born the same day, being set up under the bililights. They had the same pediatrician, so I asked her how Aidan's numbers were. She told me they were a bit high, and he would be going under the lights, too. She added that had he been full term he wouldn't need them. Aidan was under the lights about twenty-six hours total.

Each day we tried nursing, and it never went very well. He was getting sleepier and sleepier (thanks to the bilirubin), so it was suggested he needed a gavage tube. I resisted it because I thought it was a step back. In the afternoon of his third day we tearfully agreed to it since I couldn't get him to eat and his feeds were taking too much time away from the bililights. I later wished he had had the tube from the time his IV was removed so he could have gained weight faster. Day by day his feeds increased in amount and he did better. He started to gain weight. The heat in his isolette was turned down as low as it went, but they didn't put him in a regular cot. He managed to get himself "sprung" early when he peed on his bedding during a diaper change! He was set to be moved, but the nurses were too busy to get a cot ready. The nurse decided that since his bedding was wet, she would move him. Once he was in the regular cot, "going home" seemed a possibility, not a distant event.

We continued to breast-feed, bottle-feed, and gavage every three hours, and steadily he gained weight. Sometimes he would surprise us and take a full meal from the bottle. Only the nurses were gavaging him with any regularity. We were told he had to eat all his meals himself for twenty-four hours before he would even be considered for release. Every time I checked his chart to see how he was finishing his meals. I was disappointed whenever I saw "gavage x cc's." It was not too long before I noticed the nurses were the only ones gavaging him. When his dad or I was there, he always finished!

The next day (Thursday) I went in early to be sure to catch the pediatrician. She said, "He is still being gavaged, so maybe Monday he can go home." I told her, "Only when the nurses do it. We have more time for him." She said, "Maybe Saturday then." I was a bit consoled but still kind of sad at her answer. I took Aidan and got him ready for his feed. He was used to bottling only for us, so I got my expressed breast milk ready and sat down with him. I talked and sang to him as I always did and never noticed what was happening around us. I never realized the doctor was watching us; after about ten minutes she came over and said, "You can take him home tomorrow." Those were some of the sweetest words I had ever heard! I burst into happy tears.

We struggled with breast-feeding until Aidan was five and a half months. Every time I had to top him off with a bottle. He really did prefer it. The day I quit was the day I realized I wasn't breast-feeding for him anymore, I was doing it for me. Breast-feeding was a hard dream to let go of, and if I had to do it all over again, he would have been gavaged and breast-fed; no bottles would have been introduced.

Aidan has had no complications or real delays with being a preemie, and weight-wise he had caught up by about five months. It was a rough start, but it is with pride that I wear the "Preemie Mom Badge of Honor." Our second son, Evan Matthew Armstrong, arrived safe and healthy on December 20, 1998, at exactly thirty-seven weeks' gestation. He weighed 5 pounds 5 ounces and was 18 inches long. He nurses like a champ, and Aidan has adjusted very well to being a big brother!

UNCONDITIONAL LOVE:
ZAK'S STORY

by Bert Edens

Bruce B. Brown, Jr., M.D., who delivered Zak and his younger brother, Josh, died in a plane crash on January 16, 1999. He was a very dear friend, and it was a horrible shock. Zak's story is dedicated to his memory.

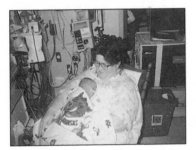

Zak with his mom, Jann Edens.

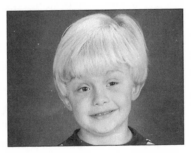

Zak in kindergarten.

"I'm sorry, but there's something wrong with the amnio."

With those words our dream pregnancy was turned upside down. My wife, Jann, was four months pregnant, and due to maternal age, her doctor had wanted her to have an amniocentesis to rule out various forms of birth defects. Even with the various risks, we never really considered the possibility of problems. Everyone wants to have a normal pregnancy, and we were certainly no exception. Jann had also had a previous miscarriage, and we were hoping this pregnancy would be a solid one.

Jann got the phone call from a nurse at work and called me in tears to say we needed to see the doctor immediately in his office. We were fortunate to have a workplace and supervisors who allowed us the freedom to leave on such short notice. We drove the short distance to the doctor's office, expecting the worst but not really knowing what to expect.

Jann's doctor told us very briefly that there was an additional piece of genetic material on one of the baby's chromosomes. He did not have details as to what we could expect from this chromosomal abnormality, what the chance of the baby's survival was, or any other information. He did offer us the option of terminating the pregnancy—a choice that went against his faith but had to be mentioned as a medical option. Jann and I both said no, we would keep the baby. Call it God's will, fate, destiny, or any other phrase, we did not believe in that choice. This baby was ours, and we would do everything we could to see that the child got every opportunity for life.

We also found out at this time that our baby was a boy. We certainly had no preference as to the gender of the child, but I must admit I was pleased it was a boy to do all those father-son bonding activities with. After receiving this information, we left almost immediately for Little Rock to see a geneticist, stopping at home only long enough to get a change of clothes. During the four-hour drive our minds raced about the possibilities, tears accompanying us all the while. This was the second of our many trips to Little Rock, so many that we eventually needed no map to get there or get around town. The first trip was for the amniocentesis, but due to my nearly losing consciousness while watching the procedure, I have no details to share.

Our visit with the geneticist was overwhelming mostly because genetics, chromosomal material, DNA, and other related medical terms were foreign to us. Fortunately, the geneticist was very kind and understanding, and helped us greatly through that emotionally charged time. It was also the start of a long professional relationship because our son continues to see her to this day. She gave us the medical option of terminating the pregnancy, which we again declined, and then began to offer details of the chromosomal abnormality and what it meant.

At that time all we knew about the abnormality was that there was additional material on chromosome eight. There are many chromosomal abnormalities they have detailed information about, including Down's syndrome, but with this one, they had very little data on what we could expect. There were few documented cases, and each involved circumstances such as a mother who smoked or drank, which made it difficult to identify the exact cause of the birth defects, delays, and so forth. The only real information they could give us was that when additional material appears on a chromosome they know little about, the baby usually dies in utero or is not able to survive outside the womb.

Armed with this minimal information and a tremendous amount of stress, the pregnancy continued. Jann worried constantly whether each day would be the one we would lose the baby. Any spotting or other problems sent her into near hysterics. I have always been very easygoing, at least externally; I usually internalize, rationalize, and then attack the problem from the best angle. I kept telling Jann I could worry enough for both of us, which I did, but it was still very hard for her.

Due to the stress of the unknown, Jann's blood pressure and glucose levels continued to rise. Her doctor continued to raise the levels of insulin she was taking, trying to keep her blood sugars under control. He also did regular ultrasounds and exams to be sure everything was going well for the baby. Unfortunately, about seven months into the pregnancy, Jann had to be put on bed rest for fear her hypertension would cause toxemia, which almost certainly would have led to fetal death and possibly even taking Jann with it. Unfortunately, the bed rest also caused more concerns about loss of income, so in some ways it helped and in other ways it didn't. Overall, I'm sure it was for the best.

Eight months into the pregnancy we went to the hospital for a late-night stress test to see how the baby would do under the stress of labor. The doctor's concern was how his heart would react to the increased stress of labor. Once we got the baby to hold still long enough, they got the monitor hooked up to Jann and began listening to his heartbeat. Little by little they increased the pitocin, which intensified Jann's contractions. Every time her contractions strengthened, the baby's heart rate bottomed out.

After being disconnected from the pitocin drip and waiting a while, Jann's doctor came in and said we were doing a stat C-section. Needless to say, we were floored. Fortunately, we already had an overnight bag packed, so I ran home to get that while Jann called our bosses and let them know what was going on. They were already starting to prep her for surgery. It was a chaotic environment, and I didn't get to see the end of the Arkansas Razorbacks basketball game I had been watching—but I will always remember the date they played their final game in their old arena.

Even though Jann and I had been through all the childbirth and C-section classes, I wasn't allowed to be in the operating room for the C-section. The doctor sympathized with me but said he would need all the available space for medical personnel, and should anything go wrong, he didn't need a hysterical father on his hands. His point was valid, but I still wasn't very happy about it.

While Jann was in surgery, I was dressed in greens and pacing in the recovery room. They definitely had to rewax the floors the next day. It seemed to take forever, but I know it was only about forty-five minutes total. I paced the whole time. Being a computer professional employed at this hospital, I kept fiddling with the workstation in the recovery room, more to pass the time than anything. After looking at it for thirty minutes or so, I couldn't handle looking at an obviously incorrect label on the front of the printer, so I changed it from "fast forward" to the correct "form feed" for the FF button. I was doing anything to keep me from thinking about Jann and the baby.

At about 11 P.M. I heard a weak baby cry and knew our son had arrived. A couple of nurses stopped by quickly to show him to me and asked if I wanted to go to the nursery with the baby. I told them that he was in good hands and my presence wouldn't help him any, so I waited for Jann to go into recovery. It was more important that I be there for her. As the nurses headed to the nursery with my son, my only thought was that comedian Robin Williams was correct: Newborn babies do look like midgets dipped in motor oil. I had to smile to myself. Sick child or not, we had a son. Zakary Tyler Edens had made his entrance into the world.

We found out shortly that Zak's Apgar scores were very low and that he was in respiratory distress. As good as our hospital was, he needed to be taken to a children's hospital where specialists could give him the best care possible. He was born late Wednesday night, and Thursday morning they were going to fly him via helicopter.

Jann and I vividly remember them wheeling Zak into her room in an isolette; he was covered with tubes, wires, and monitors. The first time we touched him, we each got to reach into the isolette to touch his hand. They left shortly after that for the children's hospital.

After a long night in which neither of us got much rest, even though Jann had the benefits of some painkillers, I decided it would be best if I rested for a day before traveling to the children's hospital to be with Zak. As tired as I was, I didn't need to be on the road for four hours by myself. It was definitely a difficult decision, but I knew it was for the best.

Thursday was a blur of visitors and well-wishers. We wanted to rest but knew our friends and family wanted to express their concern. I just wanted the time to pass quickly so I could be with our son, and Jann, having been up walking since a few hours after the surgery, had a twofold purpose: heal faster so she could travel and find some way to make the pain stop.

Finally, Friday morning arrived, and I hit the road for the long trip, bringing a large selection of music to help pass the time. As it was, the majority of my time was spent listening to Queen's "Silent Lucidity," which tells the story of a father standing over his son's crib, promising to always look after him. The song brought lots of emotions to the forefront, and to this day it remains a song deeply and emotionally integrated with Zak's birth.

Arriving at the children's hospital, I had to attend to all the admission and financial paperwork, which was the last thing I wanted to do. I then checked in at the ICU waiting room, where many parents stayed so they could be close to their children. It was for parents of children in the Neonatal Intensive Care Unit, where Zak was, and the Pediatric Intensive Care Unit, which was for older children. After getting settled in and getting a locker, I was finally able to see Zak.

I had worked in a hospital for almost eight years before Zak was born, and this helped tremendously in coping with what I encountered. After scrubbing and cleaning up thoroughly and donning a gown, I went into the NICU and was presented with a large room occupied by over thirty babies, all in very serious condition. It was overwhelming even though I had not yet seen Zak.

When I finally did see him, it took me a minute to compose myself and to accept all the wires, tubes, and monitors connected to him. He was in a bed warmer, with a bilirubin light positioned next to him to reduce his bilirubin levels. Across his head was a strip of gauze that fastened to the blanket beneath him with safety pins; the gauze protected his eyes from the harmful rays of the bililight and also prevented him from rolling around. A nasal cannula fed oxygen into his nose. He was also connected to a pulse oxymeter to measure the levels of oxygen in his blood. Various IVs were in an arm and a leg, and since they had run out of limbs, his scalp was shaved and an IV was placed there. Only one leg had been left undisturbed, and that heel was used for doing blood draws.

Sitting next to him, I let the nurse on duty explain all the paraphernalia and their purposes as I lightly caressed his back. I wasn't able to hold him because of the leads and such, so this was the closest I could get to him. It was many hours later before I convinced myself I needed to get something to eat and go to the restroom. A great fear that something would happen while I was gone was ever present, and it took a long time for me to overcome it. Even though I could have done nothing for him if something went wrong, there was still guilt associated with my leaving.

I knew it would be several days before Jann would be able to travel because she was still recovering from her surgery. During the next five days I spent almost all my waking hours next to Zak's bed, with only an occasional trip to the cafeteria or outside for a mental break. I also started a journal of my emotions and thoughts during this time, which I intend to present to Zak when he is older. When not next to Zak, which was normally during the shift change when the nurses informed one another about the patients' conditions, I spent time in the cafeteria, looking at the capitol, and making journal entries. Writing down what I was going through certainly helped me cope with the emotions, fears, and uncertainty surrounding my visits with Zak.

As a voracious reader I had purchased several new books, all with a vampire theme, before making the trek to the children's hospital. During those five days I read three of those books, almost all of them out loud beside Zak. It was slower reading, but it helped me, and I have no doubt that it helped Zak because it allowed him to hear my voice almost continuously. He has always been a "daddy's boy," and those five days were almost certainly the critical bonding period.

Reading out loud also had an interesting side effect that I wasn't aware of until I came back early from a break and the nursing staff change was still in progress. I was surprised and amused to find the nurse going off duty telling her replacement what had happened in the story I was reading to Zak. I never realized I was entertaining more than my son and myself.

When Zak was six days old, he was finally upgraded to a more stable condition, and I was allowed to hold him. I never realized how difficult it was to be near him without being able to hold him until I was finally allowed to do just that. Flooded with emotions, I almost began to cry and had to resist the urge to hold him tightly to my body. While his condition was improving, he was still very sick, as the plethora of leads and IVs still connected to him indicated. The nurse on duty took a Polaroid of us, and it has been proudly displayed on my desk at work since, a reminder of just how far Zak has come in his almost six years.

The next day Jann was permitted to travel by her doctor, so I returned home to get her. I don't believe we spent more than an hour at my mother-in-law's house, where Jann had been staying since her discharge from the hospital, before we were back on the road again. Both of us were anxious to be with Zak, especially Jann who had been away from him those first seven days. We couldn't have made more than one stop the entire four-hour trip.

When we arrived at the children's hospital, Jann was able to hold Zak almost immediately upon her arrival in the NICU, and I know this helped her tremendously. I had been able to be near him and relayed a lot of information to her via phone, but of course it wasn't the same as being there and holding our son. While I nearly cried when holding Zak for the first time, Jann definitely got misty.

It was terrific having the whole family together for the first time even if wasn't under the best of circumstances. We continued our routine, taking turns with Zak or going in together, trying to be there for him and hoping he got better soon.

Late that same night, while I was asleep in the waiting room, Jann went in to see Zak, only to find they were coding him for a heart problem. Jann expected them to rush her out, but they just sat her down and explained everything they were doing and why. They told her Zak's heart was racing, and the regular medicines and injections did not return it to its normal rhythm. The only remaining option was to stop his heart and restart it. The downside was the chance his heart would not restart. Jann left to get me, but when we came back, they wouldn't let us into the NICU. We received no explanation.

Jann and I went to the chapel and waited, not really knowing if something else had gone wrong. It seemed like forever, but it was actually only about forty-five minutes—without a doubt the longest forty-five minutes of our lives.

We found out that due to the large amounts of insulin Jann had taken to control her blood sugars, the upper chambers of Zak's heart had more muscle mass than the lower chambers, and this eventually caused an irregular rhythm. He was placed on some heart medication for about six months, then removed from it once his heart rhythm was normal and his heart had compensated for the size difference.

A couple of days after that cardiac episode Zak was moved to what the children's hospital called "feeder row," a circle of babies surrounding the more critical babies in the center of the NICU. The babies in feeder row were more stable and were able to take milk or formula from a bottle or spoon rather than having it put directly into their stomach by tube. The nurses said this was a good sign, and it certainly was a spirit lifter for us.

One of the things we found out about Zak during an MRI done in the last few days of his stay in the children's hospital was that he did not have a corpus callosum, the bridge of nerves connecting the two hemispheres of the brain. This caused problems with communication between the two hemispheres. We also learned via the same MRI that the ventricle in the left hemisphere was enlarged. The portion of the brain that it took up was dedicated to speech, so he would probably have developmental delays in his speech, which he did.

Finally, after being in the NICU for twelve days, Zak was discharged from the children's hospital and sent by ambulance to the hospital where he was born. We had asked if either Jann or I could ride with him, but they told us we couldn't. So we started back early, knowing he would be there sometime later the next day. Fortunately, with our connections inside the hospital, we were able to keep track of when the ambulance was expected to arrive because our emergency room was updated on its estimated arrival time.

Zak stayed at the hospital in isolation for two more days, mostly to try accommodating him to taking formula from a bottle. The doctors and nurses wanted to be sure there would be no problems with malnutrition once he was home. Those two days seemed to take forever, mostly because we knew we were very close to being able to take him home.

Fifteen days after Zak was born we finally got to leave the hospital. We were so excited that he was finally ours, although we were understandably scared because of the problems he had during his first two weeks of life. Most first-time parents have enough anxiety just being parents; it seemed to be magnified because of all the concerns for Zak's health. Still, we left and proudly took him out for his first public appearance: Wal-Mart.

For the first few months of Zak's life we continued on as most parents do with a new baby: adjusting to erratic or nonexistent sleep schedules, dealing with messes at both ends of the baby, trying to help the baby prosper, and many other tasks. We also made regular trips back to the outpatient center of the children's hospital to see neurologists, cardiologists, and geneticists, in addition to the regular visits to the pediatrician.

When Zak was about three months old, a coworker asked me how I was adjusting to parenthood. I replied that it was fine, but the 3 A.M. wake-up calls were getting under my skin. With that, a nick-

name was born for Zak: Chigger. He always answered to that nick-
name and probably always will. Most friends and family who have
known our family through the Internet have known him as Chigger.
It was a way of being sure he was not confused with any other
Zakary, even with our unusual spelling.

As the years have passed, we have learned a lot about Zak's chromosomal abnormality even if we don't have all the answers. It has
now been identified as tandem duplication of chromosome 8p. No
syndrome has been applied to that particular abnormality, so that is
how we always refer to it. The genetics professionals at the children's
hospital have been wonderful and tried very diligently to find more
information about Zak's situation. About three years ago we were
presented with some journal articles that detailed studies of patients
with chromosome 8. While not all of them applied to Zak, those
that did had some of the same facial features and diagnoses as he did:
high forehead and cheeks, slightly sunken eyes, enlarged head, developmental delays in speech and physical areas, and several others.
In many ways, when we looked at the pictures of the patients in that
journal article, it was like looking at our son.

We also learned there was nothing we could have done to prevent the chromosomal abnormality. It was something that happened
at germination. There was almost no risk for the same thing happening again should we decide to have more children later, which
we did. There was a 50 percent chance that Zak could pass it on to
his children and also a percentage of a chance that he could be sterile, based on the case studies. The genetics professionals at the children's hospital have continued to follow Zak every two years and
will continue to do so until he is eighteen.

Even though we started with a chromosomal abnormality, respiratory distress, and a short-term cardiac problem, we have dealt with
many other situations over the years, too. We have seen audiologists
to verify that inadequate hearing did not cause his speech delays.
Also related to the speech delays, Zak saw a maxillofacial surgeon to

be sure that improper speech patterns were not being caused by a cleft palate. The final decision was that his speech delays are based almost solely on neurological problems.

We also saw a pediatric neurosurgeon for several years, concerned that Zak's hydrocephaly and macrocephaly would eventually lead to a shunt. We were fortunate that it never did, and he was eventually discharged from their care. At one point his head size had increased significantly, and he had an MRI to look for pressure on the brain caused by the hydrocephaly. The neurosurgeon, who did not specialize in children, read the MRI and said there were no significant problems, so we did not pursue any corrective action. When we followed up with a pediatric neurosurgeon six months later, he looked at the same MRIs and decided that if he had seen Zak at that time, he would have inserted a shunt. As it was, the hydrocephaly had corrected itself, and a shunt was no longer necessary. It was ironic how that worked out. Had we seen a pediatric neurosurgeon the first time, an unnecessary procedure probably would have been performed on Zak.

At about five years of age, during a genetics follow-up, of all things, Zak was diagnosed with an irregular heartbeat, specifically a preventricular contraction (PVC.) This meant that one of the lower chambers of his heart was firing too often, causing an irregular rhythm. The primary concerns about this problem were that too many consecutive PVCs could trick the heart into establishing a new, faster rhythm, and the additional beat was not allowing the heart to compress properly, which could lead to circulatory and oxygen distribution problems.

When he was diagnosed with the PVCs, an EKG was performed to verify that the additional beats were indeed there. Shortly after that Zak had a twenty-four-hour monitor to record all of the heart's activity. The pediatric cardiologist was looking for consecutive PVCs as well as the total number of PVCs during that time period.

Another heart monitor was used three months later. The number of PVCs during the period had increased significantly, almost doubling. The cardiologist then started Zak on some heart medication, hoping to regulate the arrhythmia. Unfortunately, the heart medication also caused Zak to be extremely tired every other day. Since a fair amount of these tired days fell during the school week, we became concerned not only about Zak's quality of life but about his education. Several weeks later, following the use of another heart monitor where the number of PVCs had decreased, we changed his heart medication. That seemed to make a difference in his alertness. We do not yet know whether the PVCs have changed since the heart medication was altered.

An interesting symptom that arose about the time Zak began taking heart medication for the PVCs was his tendency to fall for no reason. After testing, poking, and prodding, the pediatrician determined the problem was with Zak's left hip. An orthopedic surgeon was unable to find anything definite even after doing a bone scan and testing for leukemia, so he referred us to a pediatric orthopedic surgeon. This meant yet another trip to the children's hospital where we have been countless times in almost six years. The pediatric orthopedic surgeon did more poking and prodding and bending and pushing, but was unable to determine the cause of the problem. Tests for early signs of muscular dystrophy were negative.

About the time we changed Zak's heart medication, the hip problems stopped. I had read on the Internet that one of the side effects of his first heart medication for the PVCs was joint pain, so it was possible that the heart medication caused the pain in his hip and made him fall due to his lack of strength and balance. Without knowing for sure what the cause was, we were just happy to see it stop.

One of the best things we ever did for Zak was to enroll him in a medical day care (available in many larger medical centers) where they could provide physical, occupational, and speech therapy for him on a daily basis and also help with his early childhood development. He was in this day care from about eighteen months of age until he started kindergarten at five and a half. Their intervention and involvement, combined with our learning what to work on when Zak was away from day care, helped him develop as much as he has. It is a testament to what loving and caring professionals can do with children whose parents are totally committed to their well-being.

The list of specialists Zak has seen over the years reads like the directory of a midsize hospital: pediatrician, pediatric cardiologist, neurosurgeon, pediatric neurosurgeon, geneticist, physical therapist, occupational therapist, speech therapist, social worker, pediatric psychiatrist, dentist, audiologist, ear, nose, and throat specialist, orthopedic surgeon, pediatric orthopedic surgeon, maxillofacial surgeon, ophthalmologist, pediatric ophthalmologist, and various others.

The list of procedures he has undergone reads about the same: MRI, X ray, CT scan, EKG, cardiac ultrasound, eye exam, hearing test, dental exam, hard palate exam, psychological exam, therapies of all kinds, countless blood tests, and evaluations of all varieties.

The constant over the last six years has been that we were always aggressive when it came to Zak. Anything that could possibly be a problem, an alternative, a solution, or even just a wild guess was attacked and either identified and acted upon or discarded. The only thing we have not done with Zak is not acted at all. We would rather have made a mistake trying than not try at all.

Today Zak is a very happy five-year-old boy. He is thoroughly enjoying kindergarten, which he affectionately refers to as "the big school." The elementary school he attends is fabulous in working his therapies into his daily activities while allowing him to remain in the primary classroom the majority of the day. We believe that Zak needs to be with children who are not special needs as well as with those who are. He needs to hear normal speech patterns, see typical, age-appropriate behavior, and be challenged to do the things his peers are doing. Zak is passing those tests with flying colors.

Zak also has a younger brother, Josh, who is two years old. When Jann got pregnant with Josh, we were concerned about the impact a sibling would have on the time and effort we would be able to provide Zak. We haven't doubted the decision since Josh was born.

The two boys are typical brothers, fighting as much as loving, but each is constantly learning from the other. Having a younger brother who is capable at two of things he is not capable of at five has pushed Zak even harder. Seeing things that Josh can do, Zak wants to prove he can do them, too. At the same time, the intense attention we give Zak with his learning has helped Josh become exposed to many things earlier than other kids might have been. Ironically, this will probably lead to having one child in special education and another in honors programs.

With all the problems Zak had before, during, and after birth, we have never regretted our decision to follow through with the pregnancy. There have been many discouraging times in the last six years, but every time we look at our older son, we realize we made the right decision. No matter how depressing or dark times may appear, no matter how discouraging the situation may be, things do get better and times do change. We need only look at where Zak is today to know this is true. We wouldn't have it any other way.

GLOSSARY OF COMMON
TERMS OF PREMATURITY

A

alveoli: tiny sacs in the lungs where oxygen and carbon dioxide are exchanged with the bloodstream.

anemia: an abnormally low number of red blood cells, which carry oxygen to tissues.

anomaly: a malformation of a part of the body.

antibiotics: drugs that kill bacteria or interfere with their ability to grow and spread.

antibodies: proteins produced by the body to fight harmful substances such as viruses and bacteria that have entered the bloodstream.

aorta: the artery leading from the heart that supplies oxygenated blood to the body.

antiphospholipid antibodies (APA): their presence indicates that an abnormal autoimmune process will likely interrupt the ability of the phospholipids to do their job, putting a woman at risk for miscarriage, second trimester loss, intrauterine growth retardation (IUGR), and preeclampsia.

APA: antiphospholipid antibodies. A large group of antibodies that cause many blood vessel and clotting problems during pregnancy.

antiphospholipid antibody syndrome (APLS): an immune disorder characterized by the presence of abnormal antibodies in the blood associated with abnormal blood clotting, migraine headaches, recurrent pregnancy losses (repeat spontaneous abortions), and low blood platelet counts.

apnea: the absence of breathing for longer than fifteen or twenty seconds.

Apgar score: a number ranging from 0 to 10 that indicates a baby's physical condition immediately following birth and then again five minutes later.

arterial blood gas (arterial stick): a sample of blood taken from an artery to measure its oxygen, carbon dioxide, and acid content.

arterial catheter (indwelling arterial catheter): a thin plastic tube placed in an artery to give nutrients, blood, and medications, and to withdraw blood for testing.

artery: any blood vessel leading away from the heart. Arteries carry oxygenated blood to the body tissues (with the exception of the pulmonary artery, which carries nonoxygenated blood to the lungs from the heart).

ASD: atrial septal defect. A hole in the septum, the wall between the atria, the upper chambers of the heart. ASDs constitute a major class of heart formation abnormalities present at birth (congenital cardiac malformations). Normally, when clots in veins break off, they travel first to the right side of the heart and then to the lungs, where they lodge as an obstruction (embolus). Once in the arterial circulation, a clot can travel to the brain, block a vessel there, and cause a stroke.

attending physician: the doctor in charge of the NICU who assumes primary responsibility for the infant's medical care. Many times this position is rotated between physicians, each one taking a month at a different hospital.

audiologist: a person trained in the assessment of hearing and hearing loss and able to determine the cause and degree of loss. The audiologist is not a medical physician.

B

bacteria: single-celled organisms that can cause infection and disease.

bagging: a procedure used to temporarily help a baby to breathe. A small mask is placed on the infant's face and an air bag is compressed, giving the baby air and/or oxygen.

bililights (phototherapy): lights used to treat jaundice.

bilirubin: a substance, yellowish in color, that is produced when red blood cells break down. The skin may take on a yellow tint (jaundice). Large quantities of bilirubin may cause a form of brain damage.

blood gas: a sample of blood taken from an artery to measure its oxygen, carbon dioxide, and acid content.

blood pressure: the pressure exerted by blood against the walls of the blood vessels. This pressure causes blood to flow through the veins and arteries. There are two numbers given during a reading of blood pressure. The first number (also called the top number) is the systolic pressure, which tells the pressure exerted when the heart contracts, sending blood to the body. The second number (the lower number) is the diastolic pressure, which tells the pressure exerted between heartbeats.

blood type: there are four blood types: O, A, B, and AB. Blood types are classified according to the absence or presence of certain proteins. Blood is also classified as Rh positive or Rh negative, indicating presence or absence of the Rh factor.

BPD: these initials stand for bronchopulmonary dysplasia. This condition is also known as chronic lung disease. It is typically induced by long-term respirator use that damages the bronchioles.

bradycardia, or "brady": a heartbeat rate that in an infant is below 100 beats per minute.

brain bleed: hemorrhaging into some part of the brain.

Braxton-Hicks contractions: these "practice" contractions occur at various times during pregnancy but can increase in intensity during the last month. They happen at random and are typically not painful—some women do not even notice them. They do not dilate the cervix, as "real" contractions do.

BRM: an abbreviated term for breast milk.

bronchial tubes: the tubes that lead from the windpipe (trachea) to the lungs.

bronchitis: an infection or inflammation of the bronchial tubes.

bronchopulmonary dysplasia (BPD) or chronic lung disease (CLD): a condition marked by respirator-induced lung and bronchiole damage.

C

calcium (Ca): a mineral element that aids skeletal development and contributes to the good health of the nervous, cardiovascular, and muscular systems.

Candida albicans (monila): a fungus known to cause yeast infections such as thrush.

candidial sepsis: yeast infection of the bloodstream causing systemic problems (like low blood pressure).

capillaries: very small blood vessels that remove waste from and provide oxygen and nutrients to body cells.

carbon dioxide (CO_2): a gaseous bodily waste product transported via the bloodstream and exhaled by the lungs.

cardiology: medical discipline focusing on the heart and circulatory system.

cardiopulmonary resuscitation (CPR): manual procedure for restarting or maintaining a person's breathing and heartbeat.

catheter: a thin tube used to drain or administer fluid.

CAT scanner or CT scanner (computerized axial tomography): a computer-controlled X-ray machine capable of capturing cross-section images of body tissues.

CBC: an abbreviation for complete blood count. A test to determine the number and types of cells in the blood. The CBC is a test to check for infection.

central line: an intravenous line threaded through the vein until it comes as close as possible to the heart.

central nervous system (CNS): the spinal cord and brain.

cerebral palsy (CP): difficulties with coordinated movements that occur as a result of brain damage.

charge nurse: also called the "shift nurse"; this nurse is in charge of the unit's nurses for a certain time period.

chest tube (ct): a tube that has been surgically inserted in the chest wall to suction away air and allow a collapsed lung to re-expand.

CLD: an abbreviation for chronic lung disease; also called bronchopulmonary dysplasia.

CMV: cytomegalovirus is a common virus that infects people of all ages. Most infections with CMV are "silent," meaning the person infected has no signs or symptoms. However, CMV infection is considered a significant public health problem because it can cause disease in unborn babies and in people with a weakened immune system.

colostomy: an opening created via surgery to allow the colon (lower part of the large intestine) to empty its contents directly through the wall of the abdomen.

complete blood count: a test conducted to count the number and types of cells in the blood; the CBC may be used to check for many things including infections.

congestive heart failure (CHF): inability of the heart to act and perform efficiently because of circulatory imbalance.

corrected age or adjusted age: the age a premature baby would have been if born on her due date. Example: A baby is ten months old (according to her birth age) because she was two months premature; her corrected age would be eight months.

CP: abbreviation for cerebral palsy.

CPAP *(continuous positive airway pressure):* pressurized air that is delivered to a baby's lungs to keep them expanded while inhaling and exhaling. The air is sometimes accompanied by extra oxygen.

CPR: abbreviation for cardiopulmonary resuscitation.

cultures: tests that are performed as a part of a septic workup.

D

desaturation or desating: a decrease in the desired amount of oxygen in the bloodstream.

dexamethasone: a steroid sometimes used following a brain injury to help reduce swelling in the brain.

Dilantin (phenytoin): a drug often used to control seizures.

Down's syndrome: an abnormality in the chromosomes that is characterized by varying degrees of mental retardation and physical malformations.

E

echocardiogram (echo): a noninvasive procedure in which a picture of the heart is produced by the echo of ultrasound waves that have been directed through the chest.

edema: puffiness or swelling caused by fluid retention in the body tissue.

EEG (electroencephalogram): a test that tracks the electrical impulses of the brain.

EKG (electrocardiogram): a test that tracks the electrical activity of the heart.

electrodes: an apparatus attached to adhesive pads that are placed on the body to conduct electrical impulses of breathing motions and heartbeat to a monitor.

endotracheal tube (ET tube): a skinny plastic tube inserted in the windpipe (trachea) to deliver air or oxygen to the lungs.

epilepsy: periodic convulsions or seizures caused by a disorder of the nervous system.

esophagus: the tube that carries food from the mouth to the stomach.

exchange transfusion: a blood transfusion in which the baby's blood is removed in small quantities while simultaneously being replaced with the same amounts of donor blood. Oftentimes this is done to dilute harmful amounts of bilirubin.

extubation: removal of the endotracheal tube.

F

fine-motor skills: the ability to coordinate the small muscles such as those of the hand.

fontanel: the space between the unjoined sections of the baby's skull that is often referred to as the "soft spot."

full term (FT): a reference to a baby born at some point between the thirty-eighth and forty-second weeks of gestation.

G

gastrostomy: an opening in the abdominal wall created via surgery to provide nutrition straight to the stomach when the esophagus is injured or blocked, or to provide proper drainage after abdominal surgery is performed.

gavage feedings: feedings through a tube inserted through the mouth or nose and into the stomach.

g-button: a feeding tube inserted in the belly button.

GERD: gastroesophageal reflux disease, a disorder in which there is recurrent return of stomach contents into the esophagus, frequently causing heartburn, a symptom of irritation of the esophagus by stomach acid. This can lead to scarring and stricture of the esophagus, which can require stretching (dilating).

gestational age: the age of a baby, counted in weeks, from the first day of the mother's last menstrual cycle before conception until the baby is delivered or reaches the full term of forty weeks.

glucose: the sugar circulating in the bloodstream and being used by the body for energy.

gram (g, GM, gm): the metric system's basic unit of weight. There are 28 grams in 1 ounce.

gross motor skills: the skills, such as crawling and walking, that include coordination of large muscle groups.

H

heel stick: the method of taking small amounts of blood from an infant's heel for testing.

HELLP: hemolysis, elevated liver enzymes, and low blood platelets. A condition that usually begins with elevated blood pressure and protein in urea, progressing to severe upper abdominal pain. If not caught early, the mother and child may die.

hematocrit ("crit"): the percentage of red blood cells in the blood.

hemoglobin: a material in the red blood cells that carries oxygen and contains iron.

hemolysis: the rupturing of red blood cells.

hernia: umbilical—at the navel or umbilicus, a lump under the skin caused by a part of the intestine that protrudes through a fragile area in the abdominal wall.

inguinal—a lump under the skin in the groin area caused by a part of the intestine protruding through a fragile part of the abdominal wall.

high risk: a term referring to people or situations needing special attention and intervention to ward off sickness (or keep it from worsening), damage, or death.

hyaline membrane disease (HMD or RDS): respiratory distress caused by a lack of surfactant.

hydrocephalus: an abnormal amount of cerebrospinal fluid in the brain's ventricles.

hyperbilirubinemia: too much bilirubin in the blood.

hypertension: high blood pressure.

hypoalbuminemia: a protein deficit.

hypogammaglobulinemia: a congenital immunodeficiency disease giving low serum immunoglobulin levels.

hypoglycemia: blood sugar levels that are too low.

hysterosalpingogram: a procedure that commonly includes injection of a contrast agent into the uterus and fallopian tubes. Examination allows demonstration and radiographic documentation of the outline of the uterine cavity. It also facilitates opacification of the fallopian tubes. Because of this, it is commonly part of the workup in cases of infertility. Also used to evaluate the tubes subsequent to tubal ligation and to evaluate the results of reconstructive surgery.

I

ICH: abbreviation for intracranial hemorrhage.

ileostomy: an opening in the abdominal wall created by surgery to allow the ileus (the part of the intestine above the colon) to empty directly outside the body.

infusion pump: a pump that delivers IV fluids in small, exactly measured amounts.

intercranial hemorrhage (ICH): any bleeding that occurs in or around the brain.

intralipids ("lipids"): a white mixture of fatty acids that is usually given through an intravenous and might be coupled with TPN.

intravenous (IV): a small needle or tube inserted in a vein to allow fluids into the bloodstream.

intraventricular hemorrhage (IVH): bleeding in the ventricles of the brain.

intubation: inserting a tube in the windpipe (trachea) to allow air to get to the lungs.

isolette: an incubator or enclosed heated bed where the temperature can be regulated.

IUGR (intrauterine growth restriction): a term used to describe an infant who is small for her gestational age.

IVIG: concentrated antibody solution given to help prevent or fight infection.

J

jaundice: a yellowish tint of the skin and the whites of the eyes caused by too much bilirubin.

K

kangarooing: holding a child skin to skin. Typically the child is laid on the parent's bare chest. (Also *kangaroo care.*)

kilogram (kg): a metric unit of measurement. One kilogram is equal to 1,000 grams, or 2.2 pounds.

L

LAC: lupuslike anticoagulant. An antibody that develops during some pregnancies that is similar to antibodies found in systemic lupus. It causes increased blood clotting and increased pregnancy loss.

lactation consultant: an individual with special knowledge about breast-feeding who can assist with nursing and pumping questions and problems. In some hospitals this person is also a nutritionist or a dietician.

lactose: the sugar found in milk.

lead wires ("leads"): the wires that lead from a monitor to its electrodes.

low birth weight (LBW): a term used to describe an infant who weighs less than 5½ pounds at birth.

lower respiratory tract infection (LRI): an infection that can attack the lungs, bronchial tubes, voice box (larynx), or windpipe (trachea).

M

Medium Chain Triglycerides (MCT): a class of fatty acids. While other dietary fats supply nine calories per gram, medium chain triglycerides provide slightly less at 8.3 calories per gram. Another difference between medium chain triglycerides and other fats is that the medium chain triglycerides are more rapidly absorbed and burned as energy.

meningitis: an infection or swelling of the meninges, the membranes found around the spinal cord and brain.

mental retardation (MR): intellectual development that is limited. There are various degrees of mental retardation.

monitor: a mechanical device that records heart rate, blood pressure, oxygen saturation, respiration, and other vital signs.

N

nebulizer: a machine that humidifies air and/or oxygen that is passed to the infant.

necrotizing enterocolitis (NEC): a condition of the intestinal tract where (normally) harmless bacteria attack the intestinal wall.

neonate: an infant during the first thirty days of life.

neonatologist: a pediatrician who has gone through special training in the care of sick and premature infants. This individual is also board-certified in neonatology.

NICU (Neonatal Intensive Care Unit): the section in the hospital where premature or sick infants can be cared for and monitored.

"nippling": bottle feeding.

NPO: an abbreviation for a Latin term, *nil per os*, that means "nothing by mouth" or stop feedings.

nurse practitioner: a registered nurse with a master's degree in nursing and specialized training who, under the supervision of a doctor, can tend to certain areas of an infant's medical care.

O

oxygen (O₂): the gas responsible and imperative for supporting life.

P

patent ductus arteriosus (PDA): a "typical" situation in preemies where the fetal blood vessel that links the aorta and the pulmonary artery does not close following birth.

pediatrician: a physician with special training in the care of infants and children.

periventricular leukomalacia (PVL): a softening of the brain near the ventricles. The softening occurs because brain tissue in this area has died. PVL is thought to be due to insufficient blood flow to that part of the brain either when the baby is a fetus in the womb, at delivery, or after delivery during the first days of life.

phenobarbital: a medication used to control seizures.

phototherapy: the use of bililights to treat hyperbilirubinemia.

physical therapist (PT): a specialist who assesses and works with problems of coordination and gross motor skills.

placenta previa: a condition that may occur during pregnancy when the placenta implants in the lower part of the uterus and obstructs the cervical opening to the vagina (birth canal).

plasma: the clear liquid part of the blood left when the red blood cells have been removed.

platelets: the part of the blood responsible for clotting.

pneumonia: an infection in the lungs.

pneumothorax: an accumulation of air in the chest cavity that results from a rupture in the lungs.

preeclampsia: the physical condition of a pregnant woman prior to eclampsia. Symptoms include blood pressure greater than 140/90; persistent proteinuria (protein in the urine); and edema.

premature infants ("preemie"): an infant born before thirty-six weeks of pregnancy.

primary nurse: a registered staff nurse in charge of the principal care of several infants in the NICU.

PROM: premature rupture of membranes.

pulmonary insufficiency of the premature (PIP): respiratory distress caused by immature lungs and lack of surfactant that attacks the youngest preterm infants.

pulmonary interstitial emphysema (PIE): a situation created when bubbles of air are pushed out of the alveoli and in between the layers of lung tissue.

pulse oximeter: oximetry is a procedure for measuring the concentration of oxygen in the blood. An oximeter is a photoelectric device specially designed to respond only to pulsations, such as those in pulsating capillaries of the area tested. May be attached to the ear or finger.

PVC: preventricular contraction.

R

RAD: reactive airway disease. Implies hypersensitivity of the air passages in the lungs. Results in tightening of the airway (wheezing).

RespiGam: a medication from MedImmune to prevent respiratory syncytial virus (RSV) and bronchopulmonary dysplasia (BPD) in premature infants.

respirator: a machine used to assist with breathing.

respiratory distress syndrome (RDS, hyaline membrane disease): respiratory distress that is caused by a lack of surfactant.

respiratory therapist: an individual trained to assist in the operation of respirators and perform procedures that assist a patient's oxygen intake and breathing.

retina: the overlay of the back of the eye that receives visual images.

retinopathy of prematurity (ROP): the abnormal growth of the blood vessels of the eye, seen in many premature infants after receiving oxygen therapy.

room air: the air containing 21 percent oxygen that we normally breathe.

RSV: respiratory syncytial virus. This RNA virus is a major pathogen in the upper and lower respiratory tract in both infants and younger children. Respiratory syncytial virus manifestations include bronchiolitis, pneumonia, and croup.

S

scalp IV: an intravenous needle placed in the baby's scalp vein.

septic workup: tests performed to check for infection.

shunt: a passage made artificially between two areas of the body, usually placed to drain liquid.

spinal tap (lumbar puncture): a procedure in which spinal fluid is extracted from the lower back by inserting a needle between the vertebrae.

surfactant: the substance made in the lungs that aids in keeping the tiny air sacs (alveoli) from collapsing and clinging together.

T

tachycardia: an exceptionally fast heart rate.

theophylline: a medicine sometimes used to treat apnea.

thrush: a fungal infection of the mouth.

TPN: total parenteral nutrition. A mixture of sugar, minerals, vitamins, and proteins given via IV.

trachea: the windpipe, which extends from the throat to the bronchial tubes.

tracheostomy: a surgical opening in the windpipe created to help air flow through the lungs when there is an obstruction in the throat.

U

upper respiratory infection (URI): an infection in the airway above the voice box (larynx).

V

VACTERLS: birth defects not related to prematurity.

vein: a blood vessel that goes to the heart and carries nonoxygenated blood.

ventricle: a tiny chamber in the heart, or in the middle of the brain where cerebrospinal fluid is created.

virus: a small infectious organism that thrives in the cells of the body.

vital signs: the pulse rate, rate of respiration, and body temperature.

Y

yeast: a minuscule fungus that can cause infections.

A complete glossary can be found in *The Premature Baby Book: A Parents' Guide to Coping and Caring in the First Years* by Helen Harrison and Ann Kositsky, R.N., published by St. Martin's Press. Consult also the Web site www.onelook.com.

RESOURCES ON PREMATURITY

Books and Pamphlets for Adults

A Fragile Beginning: Parenting Your Early Baby
A Place to Remember
1885 University Ave. W., Suite 110
St. Paul, MN 55104
Toll-free: (800) 631-0973

A Special Start by Bette Flushman
VORT Corporation Tools for Early
Intervention
P.O. Box 60880
Palo Alto, CA 94306

Baby Talk by Dale Hatcher and
Kathy Lehman
Centering Corporation
1531 N. Saddle Creek Rd.
Omaha, NE 68104-5064
Phone: (402) 553-1200
Fax: (402) 553-0507

Born Early: A Premature Baby's Story by
Bo Flood, Rebecca Young (photographer), and Lida E. Smith Lafferty
Fairview Press

Caring for Your Premature Baby: A Complete Resource for Parents
by Alan H. Klein and Jill Alison Ganon
Harper Reference

Critical Issues in the Early Development of Premature Infants by Sibylle K. Escalona
Yale University Press

The Development of Infants Born at Risk by
Deborah L. Reich
Amazon.com Books
549 South Dawson
P.O. Box 81410
Seattle, WA 98108-1310
Toll-free: (800) 201-7575
Fax: (301) 346-2950
www.amazon.com

The Emotional Journey of Parenting Your Premature Baby: A Book of Hope and Healing by Deborah L. Davis, Ph.D., and
Mara Tesler Stein, Psy.D.
NICU-INK (due out in 2001)
1304 Southpoint Blvd., Suite 280
Petaluma, CA 94954
Toll-free: (888) 642-8465

"The Future of Children: Low Birth Weight" (Vol. 5, No. 1, Spring 1995) This publication is free of charge, contact: The David and Lucille Packard Foundation
Center for the Future of Children
300 Second St., Suite 102
Los Altos, CA 94022
Phone: (415) 948-3696
Fax: (415) 948-6498
www.futureofchildren.org/ibw/

Going Home: Tips from One Parent to Another
Parent to Parent of New Hampshire, Inc.
P.O. Box 622
Hanover, NH 03755

Guiding Your Child Through Preterm Development by Tim Healey
Association for the Care of Children's Health
7910 Woodmont Ave., Suite 300
Bethesda, MD 20814
Toll-free: (800) 808-ACCH

Homecoming for Babies After the Neonatal Intensive Care Nursery
Pro-Ed
8700 Shoal Creek Blvd.
Austin, TX 78758-6897
Phone: (512) 451-3246

Infants in Crisis: How to Cope with Newborn Intensive Care and Its Aftermath by Glenn Affleck, Howard Tennen, and Jonelle Rowe
Amazon.com Books
549 South Dawson
P.O. Box 81410
Seattle, WA 98108-1310
Toll-free: (800) 201-7575
Fax: (206) 346-2950
www.amazon.com

In Time with Love by Marilyn Segal
The Birth and Life Bookstore
141 Commercial St., NE
Salem, OR 97301
Toll-free orders: (800) 443-9942
Phone: (503) 371-4445
Fax: (503) 371-5395

Newborn Intensive Care: What Every Parent Needs to Know by Jeanette Zaichkin
NICU-INK
1304 Southpoint Blvd., Suite 280
Petaluma, CA 94954-6895
Toll-free: (888) 642-8465
Phone: (707) 762-2646

The Pain of Premature Parents: A Psychological Guide to Coping by Michael Hynan, Ph.D.
Amazon.com Books
549 South Dawson
P.O. Box 81410
Seattle, WA 98108-1310
Toll-free: (800) 201-7575
Fax: (206) 346-2950
www.amazon.com

Parent Resource Guide
American Academy of Pediatrics
Phone: (847) 981-6771

The Premature Baby Book: A Parent's Guide to Coping and Caring in the First Years by Helen Harrison and Ann Kositsky, R.N.
St. Martin's Press

Special Beginnings
A Place to Remember
1885 University Ave., W., Suite 110
St. Paul, MN 55104
Toll-free: (800) 631-0973

When Pregnant Isn't Perfect
by Laurie Rich
The Childbearing Family
5032 Wendover Rd.
Yorba Linda, CA 92686
Toll-free: (800) 234-7405

Your Premature Baby by Frank P.
Manginello, M.D., and Theresa Foy
DiGeronimo
John Wiley & Sons

Books for Children

Believe in Katie Lynn
by Resta Bartholomew, Md
Amazon.com Books
549 South Dawson
P.O. Box 81410
Seattle, WA 98108-1310
Toll-free: (800) 201-7575
Fax: (206) 346-2950
www.amazon.com

*Born Early: A Premature Baby's Story for
Children* by Lida E. Smith Lafferty
Amazon.com Books
549 South Dawson
P.O. Box 81410
Seattle, WA 98108-1310
Toll-free: (800) 201-7575
Fax: (206) 346-2950
www.amazon.com

The Frogs Had a Baby, a Very Small Baby
by Jerri Oehler, R.N., Ph.D.
P.O. Box 3362
Duke University Medical Center
Durham, NC 27710

Mommy, What Is a Preemie?
International Childbirth Education
Association

P.O. Box 20048
Minneapolis, MN 55420

My Brother Got Here Early
by Patte Wheat
Available free; contact:
National Committee to Prevent Child
Abuse
332 S. Michigan Ave., Suite 1600
Chicago, IL 60604-4357
Phone: (312) 663-3520
www.childabuse.org

No Bigger Than My Teddy Bear
TLC Clothing Company
P.O. Box 245
Hunt Valley, MD 21030-0245
Toll-free: (800) 755-4852
Phone: (410) 876-9071

Special Care Babies
Association for the Care of Children's
Health
7910 Woodmont Ave., Suite 300
Bethesda, MD 20814
Toll-free: (800) 808-ACCH
Fax: (301) 986-4553

Waiting for Baby Joe
by Pat Lowery Collins
Albert Whitman & Co.
6340 Oakton St.
Morton Grove, IL 60053-2723
Toll-free: (800) 255-7675
Fax: (847) 581-0039

Breast-feeding

Breastfeeding (video)
American Academy of Pediatrics
Phone: (847) 981-6771

Breastfeeding the Infant with Special Needs
by Donna Dowling
Amazon.com Books
549 South Dawson
P.O. Box 81410
Seattle, WA 98108-1310
Toll-free: (800) 201-7575
Fax: (206) 346-2950
www.amazon.com

Human Lactation Center
666 Sturges Hwy.
Westport, CT 06880
Phone: (203) 259-5995

La Leche League International
9616 Minneapolis Ave.
P.O. Box 1209
Franklin Park, IL 60131-8209
Toll-free: (800) 525-3243
Phone: (708) 519-7730

Medela, Inc.
4610 Prime Parkway
McHenry, IL 60050
Toll-free: (800) 835-5968

Nursing Your Neurologically Impaired Baby
Childbirth Graphics
P.O. Box 21207
Waco, TX 76702-1207
Toll-free: (800) 299-3366 ext. 287

Nursing Your Premature Baby
Childbirth Graphics
P.O. Box 21207
Waco, TX 76702-1207
Toll-free: (800) 299-3366 ext. 287

You Can Breastfeed Your Preterm Baby
(three videos and brochures)

Health Sciences Center for Educational Resources
Distribution Center, SB-56
University of Washington
Seattle, WA 98195
Phone: (206) 685-1186

Diapers and Accessories

Children Medical Ventures
541 Main St. South
Weymouth, MA 02190
www.childmed.com/store

Commonwealth Premature Pampers
Toll-free: (800) 543-4932

Footsteps (baby book)
Wyeth-Ayerst Laboratories Professional Services
P.O. Box 8299
Philadelphia, PA 19101-1245
Toll-free: (800) 321-2304

Komfy Ride (car seat insert)
1625 San Marco Blvd.
Jacksonville, FL 32207
www.komfykids.com

The Preemie Calendar
Tracy Graphics
Attn: Amy E. Tracy
135 Briarcrest Place
Colorado Springs, CO 80906
Phone: (719) 576-2278

Preemie Purple Heart
www.preemie-heart.com

Prematurely Yours (Baby Books and Birth Announcements)
12515 Flagg Dr.
Lafayette, CO 80026

Toll-free: (800) 767-0023
Phone: (303) 665-2498
Fax: (303) 666-0302
www.kbryant@prematurelyyours.com
www.prematurelyyours.com

Clothing

Anne's Preemie Wear
c/o Ann Long
Route 2, Fairview Dr.
Greenville, SC 29602

For a Special Baby
Pat Cotter
1682 Roxanna Lane
New Brighton, MN 55112
E-mail: cotter@winternet.com
www.winternet.com/~cotter/
preemieclothes

Itty Bitty Britches
1203 Yonkers
Plainview, TX 79072
Phone: (806) 291-0429

ML Preemie
131 E. Highway 70
Ruidoso, NM 88345
Phone: (505) 378-7142
www.preemiestore.com/preemie.htm

One Step Ahead
P.O. Box 517
Lake Bluff, IL 60044
Toll-free: (800) 274-8440
Fax: (847) 615-7236

Premiewear
3037 Grass Valley Hwy., #8200
Auburn, CA 95602
Toll-free: (800) 992-8469
Fax: (530) 823-9884
www.premiewear.com

Tiny Angels
1110 Edgewater Beach Rd.
Valparaiso, IN 46383-1112
Toll-free: (888) 681-2175
Fax: (219) 464-9325
www.tinyangels.com

Tiny Bundles
Patricia Park
11468 Ballybunion Square
San Diego, CA 92128
Phone/Fax: (619) 451-9907
E-mail: patti@tinybundles.com
www.tinybundles.com

Magazines and Newsletters

The Early Edition
www.home.vicnet.net.au/~earlyed/
welcome.htm

Exceptional Parent
P.O. Box 3000
Denville, NJ 07834
Toll-free: (800) 562-1973

Growing Child
Toll-free: (800) 927-7289

Healthy Kids
Phone: (847) 981-7944

ICU Parenting Magazine
176 Brush Creek Rd.
Irwin, PA 15642

Neonatal and Pediatric ICU Parenting
Phone: (412) 863-6641

Parents in Touch
Neo-Flight
4364 Idlewild Lane
Carmel, IN 46033
Phone: (317) 255-5242

Preemie Parent Connection
c/o Paperworks
2668 State Hwy. 812
DeKalb Junction, NY 13630

Twins
Toll-free: (800) 821-5533

Zero to Three
National Center for Clinical Infant
Programs
2000 14th St., N., Suite 380
Arlington, VA 22201-2500
Phone: (703) 528-4300

Miscellaneous Articles and Information

After the Nicu
www.home.earthlink.net/~gbangs/
advice.html

Babycenter.com
www.babycenter.com

Car Seat Safety
www2.medsch.wisc.edu/
childrenshosp/Parents_of_Preemies/
carseat.html

Classic Neonatology
www.csmc.edu/neonatology/classics/
classics.html

For Parents of Preemies
www2.medsch.wisc.edu/
childrenshosp/parents_of_preemies/index.
html

Handling Your Baby
www.ozemail.com.au/~karlat/
handling.htm

Infant Massage
www.home.vicnet.net.au/~garyh/
prejune/0205.html

IUGR (Intrauterine Growth
Retardation)
www.chorus.rad.new.edu/doc/00942.html

IVH article by Dr. Doug Derleth
www.yarra.vicnet.net.au/~garyh/
arcmarch/0124.html

Johns Hopkins Pediatric Software Page
www.med.jhu.edu/peds/grabbag.html

Kangaroo Care
www.io.org/~infacto/skin.htm

Motherstuff clearinghouse
www.motherstuff.com

Pregnancy Complications News
www.mediconsult.com/pregnancy/news/

Prophylactic Post-Extubation Nasal
CPAP in Preterm Infants
www.silk.nih.gov/SILK/COCHRANE/
DAVIS/DAVIS.htm

www.ROP Page and Discussion Board
www.geocities.com/Wellesley/9641/
rop.html

Tender Touch
Melissa Thomas, M.N., R.N.
Saint Luke's Hospital
4401 Wornall Road
Kansas City, MO 64111
Phone: (816) 932-5174
E-mail: mkthomas@saint-lukes.org
www.saint-lukes.org/edu/ceu/
tendertouch/

Resources for High Risk Pregnancy
www.members.aol.com/MarAim/
bedrest.htm

Vaccine Response in Early Preterm
Infants
www.pediatrics.org/cgi/content/
abstract/101/4/642

Organizations

Active Parenting, Inc.
810 Franklin Court, Suite B
Marietta, GA 30067
Toll-free: (800) 826-0060
Phone: (404) 429-0565

Allergy and Asthma Network/
Mothers of Asthmatics, Inc.
3554 Chain Bridge Rd., Suite 200
Fairfax, VA 22030
Phone: (703) 385-4403

American Academy of Pediatrics
P.O. Box 927
Elk Grove Village, IL 60009-0927
Phone: (847) 228-5005

American Lung Association
1740 Broadway
New York, NY 10019-4374
Phone: (212) 315-8700

Association for the Care of Children's
Health
7910 Woodmont Ave., Suite 300
Bethesda, MD 20814
Phone: (301) 654-6549
Fax: (301) 986-4553

The Association of Women's Health,
Obstetric and Neonatal Nurses
700 14th St., NW, Suite 600

Washington, DC 20005-2019
Phone: (202) 662-1600

Children's Blood Foundation
333 East 38th St.
New York, NY 10016
Phone: (212) 297-4336

Cleft Palate Parents' Council
28 Cambria Road
Syosset, NY 11791
Phone: (516) 931-4252

IVH Parents
P.O. Box 56-1111
Miami, FL 33256-1111
Phone: (305) 232-0381

HELLP Syndrome Society
P.O. Box 44
Bethany, WV 26032
www.members.aol.com/lindapax/private/
hellp.html

HELLP Syndrome Webring
www.members.tripod.com/~AnderPander/
index.html

Lung Line
1400 Jackson St.
Denver, CO 80206
Toll-free: (800) 222-5864
Phone: (303) 355-5864

Maternity Center Association
48 East 92nd St.
New York, NY 10128
Phone: (212) 369-7300

National Association of Apnea
Professionals (NAAP)
P.O. Box 4031
Waianae, HI 96792
Toll-free: (800) 392-2514

National Digestive Diseases Information
Clearinghouse
2 Information Way
Bethesda, MD 20892-3570
Phone: (301) 654-3810

National Kidney Foundation
30 East 33rd St.
New York, NY 10016
Toll-free: (800) 622-9010

National Perinatal Information
Center
1 State Street, Suite 102
Providence, RI 02908
Phone: (401) 274-0650

Pediatric Orthopedic Society of North
America
6300 North River Rd., Suite 727
Rosemont, IL 60018-4226
Phone: (708) 698-1692

PROM page
www.hem2.passagen.se/prom/index.
htm

Single Parent Resource Center
31 East 28th St., Second Floor
New York, NY 10016
Phone: (212) 951-7030

Special Needs/Disabilities/ Birth Defects

American Academy for Cerebral Palsy
and Developmental Medicine
(AACPDM)
6300 North River Rd., Suite 727
Rosemont, IL 60018-4226
Phone: (708) 698-1635

American Council of the Blind
1155 15th St., NW, Suite 720
Washington, DC 20005
Toll-free: (800) 424-8666
Phone: (202) 467-5081

American Society for Deaf Children
814 Thayer St.
Silver Spring, MD 20910
Phone: (301) 588-6545

Association of Birth Defect Children
827 Irma Avenue
Orlando, FL 32803
Toll-free: (800) 313-2232
Phone: (407) 245-7035

Association for Children with Down
Syndrome, Inc.
2616 Martin Ave.
Bellmore, NY 11710
Phone: (516) 221-4700

Blind Children's Center
4120 Marathon St.
Los Angeles, CA 90029
Toll-free: (800) 222-3566

Children's Disability List (contains numerous online mailing lists)
www.comeunity.com/special_needs/
speclist.html

CP resource page
www.members.aol.com/cpparent

Federation for Children with Special
Needs
95 Berkeley St., Suite 104
Boston, MA 02116
Phone: (617) 482-2915

Hear Center
301 East Del Mar Blvd.
Pasadena, CA 91101
Phone: (213) 681-4641

March of Dimes Birth Defects
Foundation
1275 Mamaroneck Ave.
White Plains, NY 10605
Phone: (914) 428-7100

National Association for Parents of the
Visually Handicapped
P.O. Box 317
Watertown, MA 02272
Toll-free: (800) 562-6265
Phone: (315) 245-3442

National Down Syndrome Society
666 Broadway
New York, NY 10012
Toll-free: (800) 221-4602
Phone: (212) 460-9330

National Parent Network on Disabilities
1600 Prince St., Suite 115
Alexandria, VA 22314
Phone: (703) 684-6763

Support Groups

A.A.P.I. (American Association for
Premature Infants)
www.aapi-online.org/

Alexis Foundation
P.O. Box 1126
Birmingham, MI 48012
Phone: (248) 543-4169
E-mail: wbul63@prodigy.com

Association for the Care of Children's
Health
7910 Woodmont Ave., Suite 300

Bethesda, MD 20814
Toll-free: (800) 808-2224

Cesareans/Support Education and
Concern (C/SEC)
22 Forest Road
Framingham, MA 01701
Phone: (508) 877-8266

Intensive Care Unlimited (for
Philadelphia area and southern New
Jersey)
P.O. Box 563
Newtown Square, PA 19073
Phone: (215) 629-0449

Neo-Fight
4364 Idlewild Lane
Carmel, IN 46033
Phone: (317) 255-5242

NeoNatal Parents Network of
Oklahoma, Inc.
P.O. Box 720665
Oklahoma City, OK 73172-0665
Toll-free: (888) NEO-NATL
Phone: (405) 949-4130

Parent Care, Inc.
9041 Colgate St.
Indianapolis, IN 46268-1210
Phone: (317) 872-9913
Fax: (317) 872-0795

Parents Helping Parents of Intensive
Care Newborns
P.O. Box 268
Hilliards, PA 16040
Phone: (412) 641-6428

Parents of Preemies Support Group
6250 Hwy. 83/84 at Antilley Rd.
Abilene, TX 79606

www.abilene.com/armc/wcs/wcs_
preemsg.html

Parents of Prematures
P.O. Box 3046
Kirkland, WA 98083-3046

Parents of Premature Babies
(Preemie-1)
www.home.vicnet.net.au/~garyh/
preemie.htm

Partners in Intensive Care
P.O. Box 41043
Bethesda, MD 20824-1043
Phone: (301) 681-2708
Fax: (301) 681-2707

Videos

Baby Alive
American Academy of Pediatrics
Phone: (847) 981-6771

Baby Talk
American Academy of Pediatrics
Phone: (847) 981-6771

Caring for Your NICU Baby
Childbirth Graphics
Toll-free: (800) 299-3366 ext. 278

*Getting to Know Your Premature Baby from
Head to Toe*
Childbirth Graphics
Toll-free: (800) 299-3366 ext. 278

Infant and Toddler Emergency First Aid
(two videos)
American Academy of Pediatrics
Phone: (847) 981-6771

Injoy Videos (numerous videos; call or
write to request a catalog)
3970 Broadway, Suite B4
Boulder, CO 80304
Toll-free: (800) 326-2082

Introduction to the NICU
Childbirth Graphics
Toll-free: (800) 299-3366 ext. 278

ABOUT THE EDITORS

Kimberly A. Powell: When I became the mother of a premature daughter in March 1997, I found a new calling. I want to help other parents who find themselves in the similar, unexpected, yet eventually rewarding circumstance of being a preemie parent. Since my daughter's birth I have spent time visiting the NICU, engaging in online preemie support groups, and publicly speaking on the preemie experience. In June 1998, my daughter was featured and I was interviewed on local newscasts as a preemie success story. I use my daughter's success to help others by serving as a volunteer for the American Association of Premature Infants and a member of the HELLP Syndrome Society.

Professionally, I earned my Ph.D. in Communication from the University of Georgia in 1992. I am a college professor of communication at Luther College in Decorah, Iowa, teaching courses in public speaking, argumentation, and rhetoric. I have published several articles in peer-reviewed journals such as *Communication Studies*, *Communication Quarterly*, and *The Speech Communication Teacher*. I also serve as associate editor for *Communication Studies*, *The Iowa Journal of Communication*, and *Speaker and Gavel*, and as a guest editor for *Women's Studies in Communication*.

In addition to spending time with my family, I enjoy gardening, playing racquetball, and practicing tae kwon do. I earned my first-degree black belt in 1995, after which I began instructing in the local American Tae Kwon Do Association club.

Kim Wilson: In October 1993 I was introduced to motherhood when I gave birth to my son prematurely. Since his birth I have taken it upon myself to learn as much as possible about this unique type of parenting. I speak and correspond with several parents of preemies, mainly to hear their stories and help them through this difficult time by letting them know I've experienced the same roller coaster of emotions.

Secondary to being a mother I am a full-time freelance writer specializing in nonfiction personal interest, copywriting, self-help, and social expression. My work has been featured in both online and offline publications, including *Writer's Digest*. In addition to my writing I am part of the creative development team for the popular "Parenting Today's Teen" Web site (www.parentingteens.com). I'm also a member of the Police Writer's Club.

Several years ago, before I turned my attention to writing full-time, I worked in the medical and mental health profession. During this time I had the opportunity to assist in the delivery of three full-term babies, heightening my awareness of the differences between a premature birth and a forty-week gestational delivery.

When I am not writing, I can be found spending time with my son, Dustin, or my husband, George, reading, exploring the Internet, fishing, and enjoying other outdoor activities. I currently reside in New Jersey. I can be reached by E-mail at iowawriter@aol.com or at P.O. Box 4145, Hamilton, NJ 08610.

ABOUT THE CONTRIBUTORS

JANICE L. ARMSTRONG is a proud stay-at-home mom. She was a pre-school teacher for ten years before taking time off to raise her family. She and her husband, Stacy, and son live in British Columbia, Canada.

SUSIE BAKKEN-LANG lives in Decorah, Iowa. She and her husband, Kelly, have three children: Kim, Jim, and Dede. This is Lang's first published writing. She says, "When Kim and Kim asked me to submit my remark-able story about my father's premature birth seventy-seven years ago, I was very honored. The premature birth of your child or of someone near to you is the worst fear I think any parent or grandparent can expe-rience. In our family my father, our son, and grandson all were born pre-maturely."

CRAIG A. BRIGHT is director of real estate accounting for a major hotel company. His wife, Kelsey, evaluates federal government programs for the U.S. Congress. They enjoy travel, home improvement, and, above all, watching and sharing in their daughter Anna's exploits. Craig is also a very bad golfer who nonetheless really enjoys the game. Kelsey makes quilts in her spare time. The Brights live in Alexandria, Virginia, and can be reached at crbright@aol.com. Anna's home page can be viewed at members.aol.com/crbright/annapge/annahm.htm.

DEBORAH BROAD-ERICKSON is a native of Cincinnati, Ohio. She re-sides with her husband, Rijon, and daughter, Sarah, who was born in 1996 at twenty-eight weeks of gestation. Formerly a classical French hornist,

Deborah is now actively involved in educating and advocating on behalf of premature infants, children, and their families.

TRISH BROWN is the proud parent of an eleven-year-old daughter and a one-year-old preemie. She owns an exotic bird pet shop in Florida and is extremely active in her daughter's school as well as scouting. In her rare free time she can be found reading, at the gym, working in her garden, or on the computer. At the time of her son's birth there were only a couple of books available on prematurity. She would have been delighted to have had a reference book such as this.

KAREN CORK, wife to Kevin, is the proud mother of Griffin "Pickle" Harrison Cork, born due to complete placenta previa. Karen is an actor, and lives with her husband, son, and dog, Brock, in Calgary, Alberta, Canada. Karen has an online support network home page entitled "Club Previa and the Griffin Hype Site" at http://members.aol.com/nofoolkc. Karen is obsessed with and ever thankful for the Internet and spends any free time on the computer or daydreaming about Neil Diamond.

STEPHANIE AND DWIGHT DUNBAR have been married for one and a half years. Dwight is a network administrator for a small business office in Atlanta. Stephanie is a high school social studies teacher for Gwinnett County Public Schools in Georgia. Stephanie is twenty-seven and Dwight is twenty-eight.

BERT EDENS is an information technology professional in northwest Arkansas. His hobbies include reading, writing, computer programming, coaching, and working with children with special needs. He and Jann have been married since 1990 and have two children, Zak and Josh. Jann works as a communications professional and enjoys reading, camping, and spending time with her family.

GLORIA ETES was born in Chicago, Illinois, in 1942 and presently resides in Ridgefield, a small town sixty miles west of Chicago. Gloria has written poetry as a way to express her feelings and finds it a therapeutic way to get in touch with herself. "Megan's Prayer" was written for her granddaughter, Megan Redheffer, as she contemplated the gratitude her family felt for the wonderful care Megan received and thought what Megan might want to say if she could speak. When Megan is old enough to understand the circumstances of her birth, Gloria hopes she will like her poem.

CLARK T. KING (clark@kingproductions.com) is an advertising media specialist in the Detroit, Michigan, area. He is best known as the Web master of Tommy's CyberNursery Preemie Web (www.KingProductions.com/), which is one of the longest-standing preemie parent sites on the Internet. He enjoys weekends with his family and can be found building train layouts and dollhouses with the kids when he's not at the computer. He is a 1986 graduate of Michigan State University.

SANDRA D. MOORE is the wife of a minister in Greencastle, Pennsylvania. She loves to garden, read, write, and most of all see the excitement on Lauren's face when she "figures out" how to do something new. It is her hope that through the writing of her poem, other parents of premature children will understand that they are not alone in their feelings of confusion, sorrow, guilt, and joy. The Moore family Web site is at www.geocities.com/heartland/9477.

NANCY LYNN REDHEFFER lives in the Chicago area with her husband, David Fickert, and their pride and joy, Megan. Nancy has been employed as an economic analyst since 1985. She earned an MBA from the University of Illinois at Chicago in 1989. These days Nancy spends most of her free time with Megan but tries to squeeze in a little time for another passion, genealogical research, when possible. Nancy and David can often be found bicycling around town with Megan in tow.

MICHELLE RHAMES enjoys being a full-time wife and mother until her son is of school age. She has earned her bachelor's degree in English and hopes to complete her state teaching certificate in elementary education. Michelle enjoys reading, spending time with her family, and traveling. Her husband, Carl, is in the Air Force, currently stationed in Virginia. Together they are learning about what it means to be the parents of a child with special needs, and they hope to support other parents who are also on this rewarding journey. Their E-mail address is ares-1@erols.com. Trace Christopher's preemie page is www.geocities.com/Heartland/Woods/1514/.

JAYNA SATTLER is a stay-at-home mom to her two children, Travis and Brayden, and wife to Pete. They reside in Bartlesville, Oklahoma. Since the birth of her second preemie in 1997, she has become proactive in preemie and disabled children advocacy and education. Brayden's Web site can be seen at http://members.aol.com/moms2moms. Her E-mail address is Moms2Moms@aol.com.

B. LYNN SHAHAN worked full-time as an administrative assistant prior to the birth of her premature twins. She remained a stay-at-home mom until the spring of 1998 when she saw the twins doing fine in preschool and felt going back to work part-time would be fine. The things she enjoys most in life are sharing special moments with her family, flower gardening, going to antique auctions, and watching Austin and Ashli grow into two wonderful children. She has served as a Premature Baby Advocate locally in her West Virginia community and served on various committees as a preemie parent representative. But most of all, in the spring of 1997, she taught herself how to create a home page telling Austin and Ashli's story to reach other preemie parents searching the Internet for support. This home page is located at www.geocities.com/Heartland/Hills/9687 and is titled Preemie Twins Home Page.

MITCH SHUE is a senior software engineer at WebMethods, Inc., an Internet startup company in Fairfax, Virginia. Prior to settling in Virginia he spent several years in Texas, where he attended Trinity University in San Antonio. Mitch enjoys spending time with his wonderful wife, Vickie, and their two children, Mitchie and Carly, playing guitar, and reading. You can reach Mitch at www.mshue@earthlink.net.

CORI LAYNE SMITH is currently a stay-at-home mother to her three children. Since the premature birth of her child she has founded a preemie support group called Preemie Partners, which is based in Dallas, Texas. She enjoys spending time with her family and is currently a volunteer basketball coach for her eight-year-old son's team. She is also a volunteer for Sidelines, which supports mothers in high-risk pregnancies. If her life slows down soon, she'll also be returning to school for a nursing degree to use in an NICU. Please visit her premature son's Web site at www.geocities.com/Heartland/Valley/8095/ or E-mail her at corilayn@swbell.net.

Sally Stromseth and her husband, Don, live on a scenic farm near Decorah, Iowa. Daughters Sara and Mary both attend Luther College in Decorah, where Sara is majoring in English and Mary in music. Sally is the children's storyteller at the Decorah Public Library, where she works. Along with helping on the farm and being active in church, she also does custom orders out of her home in the Norwegian folk art of rosemaling.

Jan Sweeney currently works part-time in an accounting office for a convenience store chain. She loves to spend time with her son and boyfriend, Jody. Currently they live in Casper, Wyoming. Jan enjoys computer graphic art, desktop publishing, traveling, and cooking. She has published a newsletter for parents of VACTERLS children and loves helping those in similar situations. One day Jan would like to return to school and become a registered nurse and work in a pediatric intensive care unit. Please visit Noah's Web page at www.minidreams.com/noah.

Terry Tremethick lives in Sydney, Australia, with his wife, Karla, and son, Samuel. He currently works for Mission Australia as a network administrator. He enjoys swimming, riding, and playing with the joy of his life, Samuel. Terry has taken an interest in preemies since his son was born at twenty-eight weeks. The article, which proved therapeutic, was taken from his home page. More information can be found at www.ozemail.com.au/~karlat.

Susan-Adelle Wilshire Warren lives with her husband, Steven, and son, Samuel, in southern California. She teaches biology and chemistry at the secondary level and wants her students to share her love of science. She and Steve enjoy spending time with family and friends, singing together, and designing Web pages. Her favorite creation is her Web site about Miracle Sam at www.geocities.com /~vipreemie, which allows her to connect with other preemie parents.

Robin White is a stay-at-home mom in Richardson, Texas. She enjoys outdoor activities and reading. She has two sons, five and two-and-a-half-years old. She and her husband, Rodney, have been married for eight years. They hope by sharing their story with others that they can instill hope in those families going through a similar situation. Please feel free to E-mail her at Mamasbreak@aol.com.